12-lead Vectorcardiography

SIEMENS

With the compliments of
Electromedical Systems Division
Electrocardiography

12-lead Vectorcardiography

P. W. Macfarlane BSc PhD FBCS FESC FRSE
Professor in Medical Cardiology, University of Glasgow, Glasgow, UK

L. Edenbrandt MD PhD
Associate Professor, Department of Clinical Physiology, Lund University, Lund, Sweden

O. Pahlm MD PhD
Professor of Clinical Physiology, Department of Clinical Physiology, Lund University, Lund, Sweden

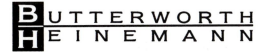

Butterworth-Heinemann Ltd
Linacre House, Jordan Hill, Oxford OX2 8DP

℞ A member of the Reed Elsevier plc group

OXFORD   LONDON   BOSTON
MUNICH   NEW DELHI   SINGAPORE   SYDNEY
TOKYO   TORONTO   WELLINGTON

First published 1995

© Butterworth-Heinemann Ltd 1995

British Library Cataloguing in Publication Data
A catalogue record for this book is available from the British Library.

ISBN 0 7506 0778 5

Library of Congress Cataloguing in Publication Data
A catalogue record for this book is available from the Library of
Congress.

Printed in Great Britain by Biddles Ltd, Guildford and Kings Lynn.

Contents

Contents

Preface

There have been innumerable textbooks on electrocardiography but fewer on vectorcardiography. This, in part, is a reflection of the complexities of recording the vectorcardiogram - at least until recently. The authors have been enthusiastic about the use of the vectorcardiogram for many years and the work presented in this short monograph reflects their interest in this area. As far as is known, this is the only book which deals with the derivation of the vectorcardiogram in a unique way from the 12-lead electrocardiogram, which is universally used. The technique has received an added boost with the relatively recent availability of microprocessor based electrocardiographs capable of printing the vectorcardiogram.

This monograph is published with the generous support of Siemens -Elema AB of Stockholm, Sweden and Burdick Inc. of Milton, Wisconsin, USA. The authors are extremely grateful to these companies for providing the guarantees which have enabled publication to proceed.

It is also a pleasure to thank a number of individuals who have assisted with the preparation of the text, illustrations and tables, namely Kerstin Brauer and Christine Edenbrandt in Lund as well as Alan Macfarlane, Stephanie McLaughlin and Elizabeth Ure in Glasgow.

It is hoped that this short book will stimulate others to learn more about the vectorcardiogram derived from the 12-lead ECG and assist them with their clinical work in relation to ECG interpretation. An elementary knowledge of electrocardiography is assumed.

Peter W. Macfarlane, Glasgow.

Lars Edenbrandt, Lund.

Olle Pahlm, Lund.

1 LEAD SYSTEMS

1.1 Introduction

The electrocardiogram (ECG) remains an important non-invasive test in the armamentarium of the physician despite increasing competition from newer investigations such as echocardiography. The reasons for the continuing interest in electrocardiography are obvious, including the fact that it is a simple, low cost, non-invasive and rapid test which provides information on cardiac rhythm, presence or absence of conduction defects, the extent of myocardial damage following an infarction and to a lesser extent, information on presence or absence of chamber enlargement. In many ways, electrocardiography has remained a dynamic subject. From the original three bipolar limb leads of Einthoven through to the currently available extensive body surface mapping systems, there has been a process of change. On the other hand, despite the present widespread availability of computer assisted methods for handling large amounts of data, the basic 12-lead ECG has still remained the most widely used electrocardiographic technique.

The ECG has recognised diagnostic limitations but more modern investigative procedures such as echocardiography are also not without problems. It has been suggested that up to 30% of echocardiograms may be technically unsatisfactory because of difficulties in recording. Furthermore, an echo recording is time-consuming and requires the use of expensive equipment. In a large teaching hospital where upwards of 30,000 ECGs may be recorded per year, even with several echocardiographs only a fraction of this number of tests can be recorded over the same period. For this reason, it is therefore important to continue to enhance the diagnostic value of the conventional ECG.

The dramatic advances in computer technology over the past 25 years have seen what formerly was almost a room full of electronic equipment being reduced in size to the equivalent of a briefcase of microchips. This has had important repercussions on all

1

branches of science including cardiology. Computer assisted electrocardiographs are now available to process an ECG in order to improve signal quality and to assist with the diagnostic interpretation. Because of the availability of advanced signal processing techniques in modern electrocardiographs, it has become possible to consider various ways of enhancing the approach to ECG analysis. The aim of this book is to highlight the renaissance of the vectorcardiogram in the light of the new computer assisted ECG machines. Not only that, but as will be seen, the need for special electrode placement to derive the vectorcardiogram can be obviated with the use of mathematical transformations which are of a trivial nature for a computer to process.

For completeness, it is necessary to review the derivation of the standard 12-lead ECG and the theory of orthogonal lead systems before progressing to a discussion on the derived vectorcardiogram.

1.2 12-lead electrocardiography

1.2.1 Bipolar limb leads

Although the first human ECG was recorded in 1887 by Waller, the leads which were used initially for diagnostic electrocardiography were the three bipolar limb leads introduced by Einthoven (1908, 1912). By using electrical connections to the right and left arms, for example, it was possible to measure the potential difference between the two – hence the term 'bipolar' lead. In the earliest systems, the patient's arms were inserted into jars of conducting solution which in turn were linked to the opposite poles of a galvanometer (Lewis, 1925). Symbolically this meant that the potential recorded by lead I was the difference between the potential at the left arm (E_L) and the potential at the right arm (E_R). In other words,

$$I = E_L - E_R$$

2

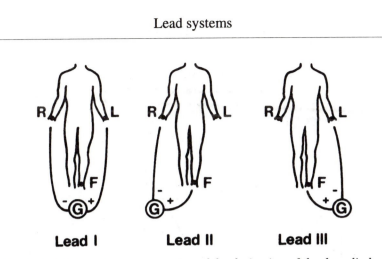

Figure 1.1 *Schematic representation of the derivation of the three limb leads.*

From similar considerations, it was possible to measure the potential difference between the left leg and the right arm to record lead II and the potential difference between the left leg and the left arm to record lead III. Symbolically,

$$II = E_F - E_R$$

$$III = E_F - E_L$$

It is a trivial matter to show that at any instant in the cardiac cycle

$$I + III = II$$

i.e. the sum of the potentials in leads I and III at any instant equals the potential in lead II. This is known as Einthoven's law. This is of importance for computer applications, indicating as it does that given any two standard limb leads, the third can be calculated therefrom. The circuitry associated with these three leads is shown in Figure 1.1. Note the polarity associated with the connections to the galvanometer denoted by G.

Einthoven et al. (1913) also introduced a model to describe the three leads (Figure 1.2). This so-called Einthoven triangle associates a direction with each of the three bipolar limb leads. Einthoven

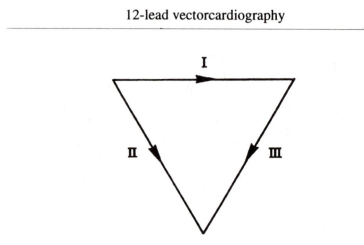

Figure 1.2 *The Einthoven triangle.*

also surmised that all of the electrical activity of the heart could be summed and represented by a single cardiac electromotive force and that the leads were measuring a component of this force in the directions denoted on the triangle. The question of components of forces will be discussed in Chapter 2.

1.2.2 Unipolar leads

In the early 1930s, Wilson et al. (1932) introduced a central terminal (Figure 1.3) which produced a relatively constant potential throughout the cardiac cycle with respect to which the potential variation at any point on the body could be measured. Wilson had met Lewis, the English physician whose early work in electrocardiography was summarised in his outstanding treatise entitled "The Mechanism and Graphic Registration of the Heart Beat" (Lewis, 1925). Both used the Cambridge electrocardiograph built in the United Kingdom and Wilson arranged for one to be shipped to Ann Arbor in Michigan where he continued his research into electrocardiography.

Because the Wilson terminal allowed measurement of the potential variation at a single point, it gave rise to the term 'unipolar lead', i.e. a lead which reflects the potential variation at a single point. Essentially, as is seen in Figure 1.3, a potential difference is being measured between a single point and the average of the potentials on the right and left arms and the left leg but because this average is essentially constant, the net effect is that the resultant waveform varies according to the changing potential at the exploring electrode, i.e. P on Figure 1.3. Mathematically, the potential at the Wilson central terminal E_{WCT} is obtained as follows:

$$E_{WCT} = 1/3 \, (E_R + E_L + E_F)$$

The new lead system allowed six additional chest leads to be recorded by agreement between American and English cardiologists (American Heart Association 1938, 1943). These lead positions are shown in Figure 1.4. The leads themselves were denoted V_1, V_2, V_3, V_4, V_5 and V_6.

Other leads which were available with the Wilson central terminal included the unipolar limb leads VR, VL, VF, i.e. leads which measure the potential variation at the right arm, left arm and left leg, respectively.

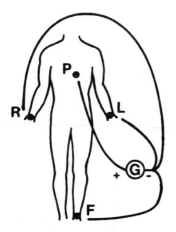

Figure 1.3 *Derivation of a unipolar chest lead using the Wilson central terminal.*

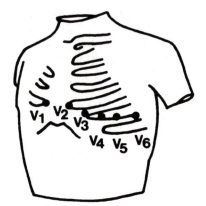

Figure 1.4 *Electrode positions for V_1-V_6.*

Mathematically,

$$VR = E_R - E_{WCT}$$

$$VL = E_L - E_{WCT}$$

$$VF = E_F - E_{WCT}$$

It follows from the foregoing equations that

$$VR + VL + VF = 0$$

Because these unipolar limb leads were of low voltage in general, they were subsequently replaced by augmented unipolar limb leads.

1.2.3 Augmented unipolar limb leads

Goldberger (1942) introduced a modification to the Wilson central terminal and this was used to amplify the voltage of the unipolar limb leads. This is best seen by reference to Figure 1.5 which shows the circuitry for the unipolar limb lead aVL. The effect of the modification is to obtain the potential difference between the left arm and the average of the potentials at the right arm and left leg.

6

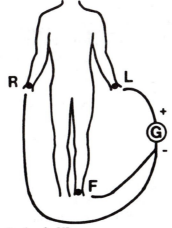

Figure 1.5 *Circuitry for lead aVL.*

Mathematically,

$$aVL = E_L - 1/2\ (E_R + E_F)$$

$$= 3/2\ E_L - 1/2\ (E_R + E_L + E_F)$$

$$= 3/2\ (E_L - 1/3(E_R + E_L + E_F))$$

$$= 3/2\ (E_L - E_{WCT})$$

$$= 3/2\ VL$$

From this it follows that the modified unipolar limb lead denoted aVL records 50% greater amplitude than the original unipolar limb lead VL and for this reason it was known as an augmented unipolar limb lead - hence the designation aVL. In a similar fashion, it is possible to design two other augmented unipolar limb leads, namely aVR (= 3/2 VR) and aVF (= 3/2 VF). It follows that at any instant in the cardiac cycle

$$aVR + aVL + aVF = 0$$

7

1.2.4 The 12-lead ECG

The various leads described above, namely, the three standard limb leads, I, II, III, the three augmented unipolar limb leads aVR, aVL, aVF and the six unipolar chest leads V_1-V_6, together constitute the 12-lead ECG. Occasionally, usually in children but not always, additional right sided chest leads are recorded. If V_3 is reflected onto the right side of the chest, then V_{3R} is recorded - similarly for V_{4R}, V_{5R} and V_{6R}.

1.2.5 Redundancy

As mentioned in connection with Einthoven's Law, there is redundancy in the standard limb leads. It also follows from the foregoing equations that there is redundancy in the augmented unipolar limb leads. In fact, it can be shown that if any two of the six frontal plane leads are recorded, then the other four can be calculated therefrom.

It is commonplace nowadays for computer assisted electrocardiographs essentially to record and store only leads I and II and V_1-V_6 although all 12 leads would be displayed, of course. Consider how aVL could be derived from I and II:

$$aVL = E_L - 1/2\,(E_R + E_F)$$

$$= 1/2\,(E_L - E_R) + 1/2\,(E_L - E_F)$$

$$= 1/2\,I + 1/2\,(-III)$$

$$= 1/2\,I - 1/2\,(II - I)$$

$$= I - 1/2\,II$$

Similarly, it can be shown that

$$aVR = -1/2\,(I + II)$$

8

and that

$$aVF = II - 1/2 \ I$$

It again follows in a trivial fashion that

$$aVR + aVL + aVF = 0$$

1.2.6 Lead display

The concept of a 'direction' for each lead was introduced in connection with the frontal plane leads I, II and III. However, in a similar fashion, a direction can be associated with the other leads aVR, aVL, aVF. These directions are obtained by drawing a line from the centroid of the Einthoven triangle to each of the vertices as in Figure 1.6. From this, it becomes possible to draw 'directions' for each of the six leads and indeed, to introduce, in a sense, a new 'direction', that of –aVR, which is intermediate to leads I and II. Mathematically,

$$-aVR = 1/2 \ (I + II)$$

This so-called modified hexaxial reference frame (Figure 1.7) can be used to discuss lead presentation.

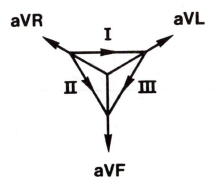

Figure 1.6 *Directions of the leads I, II, III, aVR, aVL and aVF with respect to the Einthoven triangle.*

9

For historical reasons, leads I, II and III were generally presented as a group of three leads whether recorded simultaneously or not. With the much later introduction of the augmented unipolar limb leads, another group of three leads aVR, aVL and aVF classically was displayed simultaneously beneath each other. Of course, the six precordial leads V_1 to V_6 were displayed in that sequence, even if in groups of three.

An alternative lead presentation now believed to be known wrongly as the Cabrera Format (which is commonly used in Sweden) is based on the display of the frontal plane leads in the logical sequence aVL, I, –aVR, II, aVF, III (Figure 1.8). Note that –aVR is chosen in preference to aVR. An international group of electrocardiographers has supported the more widespread use of this display format.

All of these display formats are selected very easily in a computer based electrocardiograph which can position the leads in any desired sequence (within limits!) on the output device.

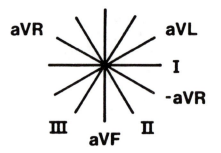

Figure 1.7 *Modified hexaxial reference frame.*

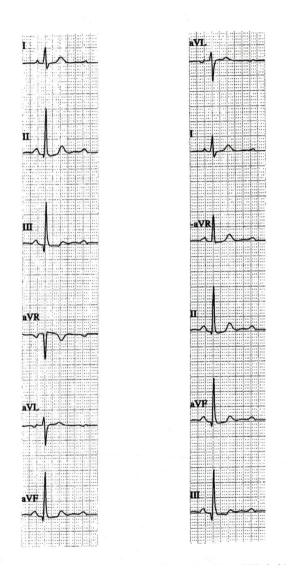

Figure 1.8 *Conventional sequence I, II, III, aVR, aVL, aVF (left) and alternative display aVL, I, –aVR, II, aVF, III (right).*

2 VECTORCARDIOGRAPHY

2.1 What is a vector?

The term vector can have different meanings but for the purposes of the study of vectorcardiography, the relevant definition states that a vector is an entity possessing a magnitude and a direction. For example, if a wind blows in an easterly direction at 10 km per hour, it could be represented by the vector in Figure 2.1a. On the other hand, if a light breeze blows at 5 km per hour in a north easterly direction, it would be represented using the same scheme by the vector of Figure 2.1b. It can be seen that the length of the vector is proportional to the strength of the wind and the direction of the vector is that of the wind.

There can, of course, be many different forces that are represented by a vector. Within the context of electrocardiography, it is the cardiac electromotive force that it is desired to represent by a vector. It was Einthoven et al. in their classic paper of 1913 who suggested that the electrical forces of the heart could be summed and represented by a single vector.

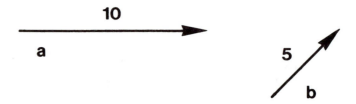

Figure 2.1 *The direction and speed of the wind represented as a vector when the (**a**) wind blows in an easterly direction at 10 km per hour (**b**) wind blows in a north easterly direction at 5 km per hour.*

2.2 Concept of resultant force

While a vector can be used to represent an individual force as shown in Figure 2.1, a series of vectors can be used simultaneously to represent a variety of forces acting together or in opposition. It is possible to use some simple mathematical techniques to calculate the resultant effect of the different forces, and it is instructive to consider an example.

Imagine that a rower sets out to cross a river. He is able to row constantly at 4 km per hour directly across the water but has to contend with a current which is flowing at a rate of 3 km per hour. This is depicted in Figure 2.2. It should be clear that if the rower consistently pulls directly across the river he will not reach the bank at a point directly opposite his starting point but will be carried some way downstream by the current. In fact, the distance can be calculated by what is known as the 'Triangle of Forces' which shows that he would travel at a net speed of 5 km per hour. The exact point at which the rower reaches the opposite bank, of course, depends on the width of the river but this can be calculated from the triangle.

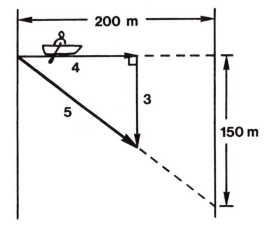

Figure 2.2 A rower crossing a river 200 m wide. For explanation see text.

For example, if the river is 200 m wide, the boat should reach the opposite side 150 m downstream on the opposite side.

The combined velocity of the boat and the current produces a resultant velocity of 5 km per hour depicted by the hypotenuse on the triangle. Conversely, it can be said that if there is a resultant velocity of 5 km per hour, it has components of 3 km and 4 km per hour at right angles to each other in keeping with Figure 2.2. Thus, there exists the concept that a resultant velocity has a component in a particular direction. The size of each component can be obtained by drawing a perpendicular from the tip of the resultant vector to a line indicating the direction in which it is desired to measure the component.

A similar concept applies in electrocardiography. Consider that in the frontal plane of the body, there is a resultant cardiac electromotive force of 2 mV acting at 45° to the horizontal, i.e. approximately similar to the path of the rowing boat in Figure 2.2. Figure 2.3 shows that there is a component of 1.41 mV in the direction of lead I. Similarly, it can be shown that there is a component of

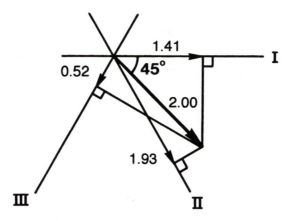

Figure 2.3 *The cardiac electromotive force and its components in the direction of leads I, II, III.*

14

approximately 1.93 mV in the direction of lead II. This estimate assumes that the equilateral Einthoven triangle is a valid model which in reality is not the case. However, the potential measured by lead I can be considered as the component of the resultant cardiac electromotive force acting in that direction in the frontal plane. It follows from Einthoven's Law that the potential in lead III would be 0.52 mV at the same instant in the cardiac cycle.

2.3 Spatial vector

Sections 2.1 and 2.2 have dealt with the 2-dimensional situation of a vector or vectors acting effectively in a plane. A more realistic situation is a force or a vector having the ability to be directed at any point in space. Figure 2.4 illustrates the concept of a spatial vector drawn within a 3-dimensional coordinate reference system with axes denoted X, Y and Z. It can be seen from the illustration that

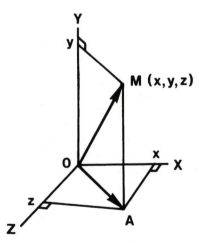

Figure 2.4 A spatial vector OM and its components x, y, z in a 3-dimensional coordinate system.

15

the magnitude of the vector can be calculated from using triangle OMA if the length of sides OA and AM can be determined. However, from the Figure, it follows that:

$$OA^2 = x^2 + z^2$$

From right angled triangle OMA,

$$OM^2 = OA^2 + AM^2 = x^2 + y^2 + z^2$$

Thus, for a point M with coordinates x, y, z in 3-dimensional space, the length of the vector OM is given by the above expression. By analogy with the 2-dimensional situation, where it was shown that a vector lying in a plane could have components calculated in any particular direction by drawing a perpendicular to that line, it can also be shown that in the spatial situation, a vector, e.g. OM, can have components in the three mutually perpendicular directions X, Y, Z. In the forward situation, if the components x, y, z can be measured at a particular instant in the cardiac cycle, then a resultant OM can be calculated. This is the basis of an orthogonal lead system.

2.4 Orthogonal lead systems

2.4.1 Theoretical considerations

The previous section suggests that if three leads can be designed to record components of a resultant cardiac electromotive force in three mutually perpendicular directions, then the problem of deriving the resultant cardiac electromotive force is solved. A considerable amount of research went into designing such lead systems over the past 50 years. The theory is detailed but a few simple concepts are worthy of discussion at this point. Further aspects are considered in 3.1.1.

Suppose that the potential measured by any electrocardiographic lead is represented by V. Then, assume that the resultant cardiac

16

electromotive force is denoted by **H** or, as it is sometimes known 'The heart vector'. Then from mathematical considerations, it can be shown that $V = \mathbf{H \cdot L}$ where **L** is the vector representing the strength of the lead being used to measure the potential. In fact, it is one of the basic rules of vector mathematics that the dot product of two vectors is a scalar, i.e. potential or voltage does not have an associated direction but only a magnitude whereas the heart vector **H** and the lead vector **L** each has its own direction. This basic rule of vector mathematics can also be expanded to the following:

$$V = H_X L_X + H_Y L_Y + H_Z L_Z$$

where H_X, H_Y, H_Z are the three components of the heart vector and L_X, L_Y, L_Z are the three components of the lead vector. From this it follows that if it is desired to measure the component of the heart vector in the X direction, then a lead should be designed that has components $(L_X, 0, 0)$. In that case

$$V_X = H_X L_X$$

If the strength L_X of the lead is known, then when the potential V_X is measured, H_X can be calculated.

2.4.2 Uncorrected lead systems

For historical reasons, it is worth noting that the earliest attempts at designing orthogonal lead systems were made on the basis of constructing leads such that lines joining the electrodes were essentially mutually perpendicular. This is most easily understood by considering the cube system introduced by Grishman (1952) (Figure 2.5). However, as experience was gained and mathematical modelling advanced, it was found that these lead systems did not accurately measure the required components.

2.4.3 Corrected orthogonal lead systems

As a result of considerable modelling, both mathematical and physical, such as using model torsos filled with conducting solution,

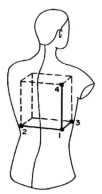

Figure 2.5 *The cube lead system introduced by Grishman (After Frank (1954a). ©American Heart Association, Dallas, Texas. Reproduced with permission.)*

corrected orthogonal lead systems gradually were introduced. The most notable and the one which is generally used wherever vector-cardiography is currently studied using an orthogonal lead system, is that of Frank (1956). This lead system is shown in Figure 2.6. As can be seen, the lead positions are different from those of the 12-lead system although the C and A electrodes are indeed close to the V_4 and V_6 positions, respectively.

Mathematical modelling showed that the following equations represent the derivation of the three potentials V_X, V_Y, V_Z.

$$V_X = 0.610\ V_A + 0.171\ V_C - 0.781\ V_I$$

$$V_Y = 0.655\ V_F + 0.345\ V_M - 1.0\ V_H$$

$$V_Z = 0.133\ V_A + 0.736\ V_M - 0.264\ V_I - 0.374\ V_E - 0.231\ V_C$$

These contributions to the individual leads from the different electrodes correspond to the resistor network also seen in Figure 2.6. The major disadvantage of using this type of orthogonal lead sys-

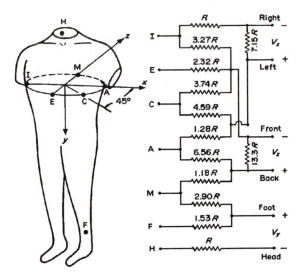

Figure 2.6 *The Frank lead system (After Frank (1956). © American Heart Association, Dallas, Texas. Reproduced with permission.)*

tem is the need to apply a completely different set of electrodes to the patient compared to that required for recording the conventional 12-lead ECG. There have been attempts to minimise the differences by doubling the C and A electrodes as V_4 and V_6, for example, and using a common left leg electrode but this still leaves four additional electrodes to be positioned on the thorax and neck.

2.5 Cardiac activation

2.5.1 Vectorial spread of cardiac activation

The concept of resultant cardiac electromotive force by now should be gaining hold. It is possible to consider the various resultant forces acting throughout ventricular depolarisation, for example. Figure 2.7a shows a series of individual vectors each of which represents the resultant cardiac electromotive force at one particular instant during the process of ventricular depolarisation. For example, the first small vector shows the initial septal activation from left to right. Note that all of these vectors are depicted in the 2-dimensional situation which in this case is the frontal plane of the body. Figure 2.7b indicates how each of these resultant vectors can be translated to a common origin and a loop drawn to connect the tips of the vectors. This loop is a form of vectorcardiogram. Indeed, the first form of planar vectorcardiogram was introduced by Mann in 1920.

2.5.2 Spatial vector loop

The previous section showed a planar loop. However, the concept of spatial vector has been introduced in 2.3 and it follows that if a resultant vector varies in magnitude and direction throughout the cardiac cycle, then it can be imagined that the tip of this vector will trace out a 3-dimensional path. This is illustrated in Figure 2.8 for the case of ventricular depolarisation, i.e. a spatial QRS loop is

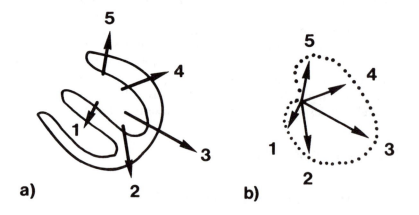

Figure 2.7 (a) *Ventricular depolarisation illustrated as a sequence of vectors, 1-5. (b) After translation of vectors to a common orgin, a vector-cardiographic loop can be constructed.*

shown. In addition, the projection of this loop onto three mutually perpendicular planes is also illustrated. The collection of three planar loop projections is known as the vectorcardiogram. While only the QRS loop is depicted here for clarity, it follows that P and T loops can also be derived.

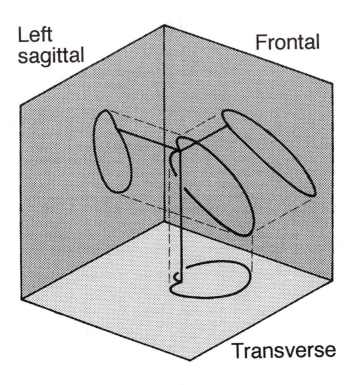

Figure 2.8 *A vectorcardiographic loop in space projected onto the three orthogonal planes.*

2.6 Vector loop presentation

2.6.1 Nomenclature

The American Heart Association committee on electrocardiography (1975) published a set of recommendations for vectorcardiographic terminology. The committee recommended that the lead Z be directed positively to the posterior thorax, although this does mean

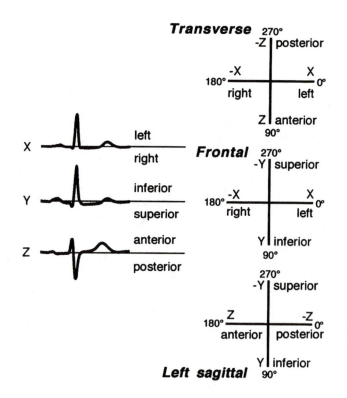

Figure 2.9 *Polarity of leads X, Y and Z and angular reference frame of the frontal, transverse and left sagittal planes.*

22

that the scalar presentation of lead Z is essentially opposite to that of lead V_2. This certainly causes much confusion when describing scalar lead appearances and for this reason, in this book, lead Z is directed positively to the anterior to be similar to V_2. Thus R_Z can be thought of in the same way as R_{V2}. Of more contention is the choice of whether to view the left or right sagittal planes, i.e. the sagittal plane as viewed from the left or right. Figure 2.9 shows the left sagittal projection. The Committee did not make a particular recommendation, but for the purposes of illustrations in this book, the left sagittal view has been chosen in keeping with Figure 2.9 so as to have a uniform collection of reference axes.

2.6.2 Display techniques

About 20 years ago the most common method of displaying the vectorcardiogram was via an oscilloscope. Pairs of leads such as X and Y were used to deflect the electron beam horizontally and vertically, respectively, and in this case, the frontal plane loop would be generated. Consider that leads X and Y are recorded simultaneously. At any instant in time, an amplitude for each lead is known, i.e. an (x, y) coordinate pair of values is available. These could be plotted simply on XY axes. If this is repeated throughout the cardiac cycle, then a complete frontal plane set of P, QRS and T loops can be generated. Figure 2.10 shows the derivation of a QRS loop in the transverse plane.

If the leads X, Y, Z are considered in pairs, then by plotting leads XY, the frontal plane vectorcardiographic loop can be obtained. Similarly XZ plots produce the transverse plane loop and ZY plots produce the sagittal plane vectorcardiographic loop. Nowadays, with the widespread availability of computer technology, these plots can be produced in a straightforward fashion. It is somewhat more complex to program a thermal writer to produce an XY display but nevertheless this is readily attainable. Thus, vectorcardiographic loops can now be produced even on small 4" paper displays or on the larger A4 writers such as are common at the bedside. An

23

illustration of a typical vectorcardiographic display from a computer based electrocardiograph is shown in Figure 2.11

It is important that vectorcardiographic loops have some indication of the speed of inscription as this can contain diagnostic information. A number of methods have been used. Conventionally, the vectorcardiographic loop has been interrupted so that time intervals can actually be measured by counting the number of dots between two points. Generally, 2 or 4 ms intervals have been used. An alternative is to produce a continuous loop and mark a number such as 1, 2 indicating 10, 20 ms etc. from the onset of the QRS complex. This is helpful but creates difficulties around the onset and termination of the QRS loop which is often the most interesting part in terms of looking for conduction problems. Either way, the direction of inscription of the loop is also of vital clinical significance. Thus,

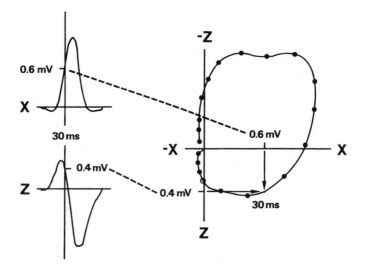

Figure 2.10 *Derivation of transverse plane loop from leads X and Z. Dots are at 4 ms intervals and the 20 ms vector is indicated with an open circle.*

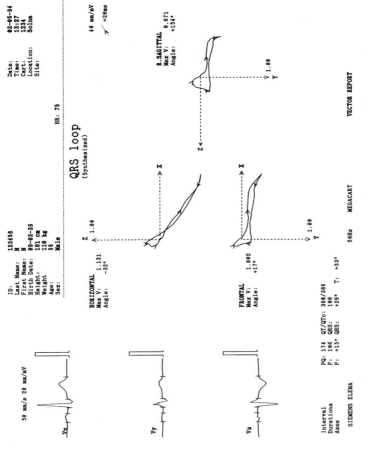
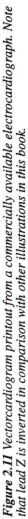

Figure 2.11 *Vectorcardiogram printout from a commercially available electrocardiograph. Note that lead Z is inverted in comparison with other illustrations in this book.*

25

if a numbering system is not used, some indication must be given to make it quite clear to the viewer in which direction the different planar loops are inscribed. With a knowledge of the theory of vectorcardiography, the experienced cardiologist can always determine the direction of inscription but it is certainly easier if this is made obvious in a good display.

In this book, loops are presented with an arrow indicating the direction of inscription. Further, black dots indicate 4 ms intervals and the 20 ms vector is indicated with an open circle.

3 DERIVED LEADS

3.1 Introduction

When computers were first used for interpretation of the ECG, there were two competing approaches. In one, the conventional 12-lead ECG was used with each lead being recorded singly (Caceres et al., 1962). In the other, the 3-orthogonal lead ECG was used by Pipberger and co-workers (1961a). At that time, research groups used physically large computer systems which were not necessarily fast, certainly by today's standard. For this reason, it was of interest to use the minimum number of leads necessary to obtain a satisfactory diagnostic interpretation. In 1961, Pipberger et al. (1961b) had shown that the 3-orthogonal lead ECG contained as much clinical information as the 12-lead ECG. The Glasgow group, for example, also confirmed this using computer assisted interpretation for both types of lead system (Macfarlane, Lorimer, Lawrie, 1971).

The 3-orthogonal lead system was quicker to use in that it required only 10 seconds of three leads recorded simultaneously as opposed to 10 seconds of eight independent leads of the 12-lead ECG recorded consecutively or even 4 x 5 seconds where the 12-lead ECG was recorded in groups of three leads simultaneously (Bonner et al., 1972). In addition, the concept of telephone transmission of ECGs was being implemented widely at that time and the 3-orthogonal lead ECG could also be transmitted more quickly than the 12-lead ECG. However, the X, Y, Z leads were not well understood by physicians.

Possibly for these reasons, Dower et al. (1980) in Vancouver had the idea that the 12-lead ECG could be derived from the three orthogonal leads X, Y, Z. In order to understand the thinking behind this, it is necessary to review the theory.

3.2 Derived 12-lead ECG

3.2.1 Frank's image space

In developing his 3-orthogonal lead system (see 2.4.3), Frank (1954b) made use of the concept of image space. This can be explained as follows.

It was shown in 2.4.1 that the potential V_P at any point P on the surface of the body or a torso model is given by

$$V_P = H_X L_X + H_Y L_Y + H_Z L_Z$$

where H_X, L_X, etc are heart and lead vector components, respectively.

If a torso model is used and the heart vector is represented by a physical dipole, it is feasible to study the potential measurements on the surface of the torso model. If the dipole is oriented in the X direction then the potential at point P is given by $V_P = H_X L_X$ because L_Y and L_Z are zero. Now, if the physical dipole is given unit strength, i.e. $H_X = 1$, then the equation reduces further to $V_P = L_X$. In other words, the X component L_X of the lead vector corresponding to the point P can be measured. Similarly, L_Y and L_Z can be obtained. Thus, the components of the lead vector L can be determined. In effect, the components L_X, L_Y, L_Z provide the coordinates of another point in space.

If this procedure is repeated for a large number of points P on the surface of the torso model, then in a similar fashion, a complete set of points corresponding to the tips of the lead vectors for the various points P will be obtained. There is, in other words, a mapping for each point P on the physical torso surface onto an imaginary or image surface determined by the coordinates of the various lead vectors L_P. This was the image surface described by Frank (1954b) (Figure 3.1).

The beauty of the image surface was that, for example, a line joining two points on the image surface corresponding to two points on

FRONTAL VIEW

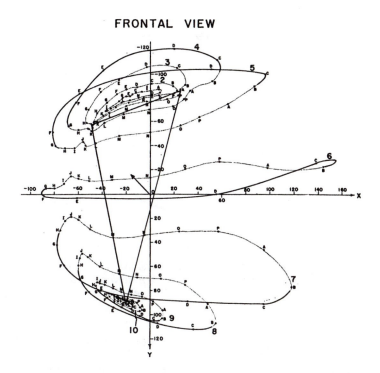

Figure 3.1 *Frontal view of Frank's image surface. Note the representation of the Einthoven triangle. (After Frank (1954b) © Mosby-Yearbook, St. Louis, Missouri. Reproduced with permission)*

the torso model would map out the actual lead direction for the bipolar lead so constructed. Thus, the magnitude and direction of the lead vector could be obtained experimentally.

In a similar way, but with a little more mathematics being involved, Frank was able to study the effect of the combinations of various potentials and derive the resultant lead vector using his image surface. A further example is given in Figure 3.2. In fact, this is an illustration of the derivation of the lead vector for lead X of the Frank lead system (1956).

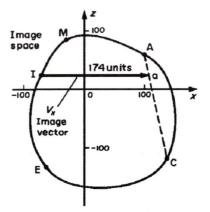

Figure 3.2 *The X lead vector in the Frank lead system constructed from Frank's image space. (After Frank (1956). ©American Heart Association, Dallas, Texas. Reproduced with permission)*

3.2.2 The derived 12-lead ECG according to Dower

In the same way as the orthogonal lead vectors can be constructed using the image surface of Frank, it is possible to study the standard 12-lead ECG. For example, by assuming that the potential measured by lead I is the potential difference between the upper right and left shoulders corresponding to the extremities of the Frank image surface, a line joining these two points in image space does indeed give the direction of the vector for lead I (Figure 3.1). If it is the case that potentials from leads X, Y and Z are available, it is then possible using the image space to construct a system whereby a percentage of each of the potentials measured by these leads is added together to produce the potential that would be measured by lead I. This can be understood perhaps by referring to the concept of resultant force discussed in Section 2.2 and in particular, Figure 2.3.

30

In general terms, it can be shown that any lead can be derived from the X, Y, Z leads using the following form of equation:

$$V_{derived} = aX + bY + cZ$$

where a, b, c are coefficients derived from the image surface.

Since lead X measures electromotive force directed to the left axilla and lead I theoretically undertakes a similar measurement, it would be expected that a derived lead I would in large measure consist of a high percentage of the potential of lead X with perhaps a small percentage of the potentials of leads Y and Z to take account of the differences in lead vector magnitude and direction between lead I and lead X. Indeed, it was shown by Dower et al. (1980) that

$$\text{lead I} = 0.632\,X - 0.235\,Y - 0.059\,Z$$

This equation applies at any instant in the cardiac cycle so that if the ECG is perhaps being sampled using an analogue to digital converter at 500 samples per second, then the calculation of lead I from the X, Y, Z leads would require to be undertaken 500 times to create one second of lead I. If the input from the analogue to digital converter is in microvolts then the output from the equation is also in microvolts.

Although the discussion has suggested a digital design for converting from one set of leads to another, it is possible to construct an analogue circuit which continuously produces the 12-lead ECG from X, Y, Z inputs (Dower et al., 1980).

The above equation for lead I was provided as an example. Similarly, coefficients a, b, c can be provided for the calculation of any of the 12 leads and these are shown in Table 3.1. These coefficients were calculated on the basis of lead Z being directed positively anteriorly. The table is presented in a 12 x 3 matrix so that the equation for each lead can be easily determined, as well as the fact that this is of convenience for subsequent discussion.

A comparison of the derived 12-lead ECG, with the actual 12-lead ECG recorded from a patient, in large measure shows good similar-

31

ity but there are nevertheless many occurrences of significant differences between the two. For this reason, the derived 12-lead ECG perhaps did not gain the acceptance that it might otherwise have achieved. The value of the concept, however, will be seen later.

Table 3.1 Coefficients for deriving the 12-lead ECG from Frank leads X, Y and Z. See text for further explanation.

	X	Y	Z
I	0.632	–0.235	–0.059
II	0.235	1.066	0.132
III	–0.397	1.301	0.191
aVR	–0.434	–0.415	–0.037
aVL	0.515	–0.768	–0.125
aVF	–0.081	1.184	0.162
V_1	–0.515	0.157	0.917
V_2	0.044	0.164	1.387
V_3	0.882	0.098	1.277
V_4	1.213	0.127	0.601
V_5	1.125	0.127	0.086
V_6	0.831	0.076	–0.230

3.3 Derived X, Y, Z leads

3.3.1 Methods of derivation

Different methods of deriving the X, Y, Z leads from the 12-lead ECG have been proposed. In a comprehensive review, Rubel et al. (1991) compared eight different published approaches and concluded that either a regression technique or a method based on the reverse of Dower's approach described in 3.2.2 provided the best solution. Other methods include, at the one extreme, using leads I, aVF, V_2 as substitutes for X, Y and Z to more complex mathematical techniques for deriving regression equations for each mapping which nevertheless are simple to apply. Each approach is discussed in turn.

3.3.2 Simple analogues

Although it is quite feasible to suggest that I, aVF and V_2 are in a sense equivalent to X, Y and Z, these leads are not mutually perpendicular, at least according to Frank's image surface. However, very similar approaches have been used. For example, Bjerle and Arvedson (1986) suggested:

$$X = 1.06 \, V_6$$

$$Y = 1.88 \, VF = 1.25 \, aVF$$

$$Z = 0.532 \, V_2 - 0.043 \, V_6$$

Marquette Electronics used the following transformation:

$$X = I$$

$$Y = aVF$$

$$Z = 0.8 \, (V_1 + V_2 / 2)$$

3.3.3 Regression techniques

If the 12-lead and the corresponding X, Y, Z lead ECG are available from a large number of patients, then it becomes feasible to use statistical techniques to calculate regression coefficients that allow the X, Y, Z leads to be expressed in the following form:

$$X = aI + bII + cV_1 + dV_2 + eV_3 + fV_4 + gV_5 + hV_6$$

This approach was used by Kors et al. (1990), who provided coefficients for leads II and III rather than I and II, e.g.

$$X = 0.58\ II - 0.82\ III - 1.27\ V_1 - 0.55\ V_2$$

$$+ 0.72\ V_3 + 1.86\ V_4 + 1.92\ V_5 + 1.53\ V_6$$

3.3.4 Matrix inversion technique

Table 3.1 expressed the coefficients for deriving the 12-lead ECG from the X, Y, Z leads as a 12 x 3 matrix. If this matrix of transfer coefficients is denoted by **T** then the equation for deriving the 12-lead ECG, **E**, from the vector leads X, Y, Z denoted by **V** can be expressed in a matrix form as follows:

$$\mathbf{E = TV}$$

By using mathematical manipulation, it is possible to turn the equation around so that the vector leads **V** can be derived from a knowledge of the 12-lead ECG. The matrix manipulation is as follows:

Let

$$\mathbf{I = N^{-1}N}$$

be the identity matrix and

$$\mathbf{N = T^tT}$$

Then

$$V = IV$$

$$= (N^{-1}N) \, V$$

$$= (N^{-1}(T^tT))V$$

$$= N^{-1}T^tE$$

The reader who has no background in matrix techniques need not be concerned about the above but will, of course, be interested in the result, namely, that each of the orthogonal leads X, Y and Z can be expressed as a linear combination of the 12 leads. For example:

$$\text{lead } Z = 0.229 \, V_1 + 0.310 \, V_2 + 0.246 \, V_3 + 0.063 \, V_4$$

$$- 0.055 \, V_5 - 0.108 \, V_6 - 0.022 \, I - 0.102 \, II$$

The complete set of transfer coefficients is given in the 3 x 8 matrix of Table 3.2 where lead Z is directed positively anteriorly.

Because the 'matrix' of values in Table 3.1 has been inverted in a sense, this approach has been called the 'inverse Dower' technique (Edenbrandt and Pahlm, 1988).

Table 3.2 Coefficients for deriving the orthogonal leads X, Y, Z from the 12-lead ECG. See text for explanation.

	V_1	V_2	V_3	V_4	V_5	V_6	I	II
X	−0.172	−0.074	0.122	0.231	0.239	0.194	0.156	−0.010
Y	0.057	−0.019	−0.106	−0.022	0.041	0.048	−0.227	0.887
Z	0.229	0.310	0.246	0.063	−0.055	−0.108	−0.022	−0.102

3.3.5 Paediatric equations

As the reader may be aware, it is common practice in recording the paediatric ECG to replace lead V_3 by V_{4R}. For this reason, the transfer coefficients provided in all of the above sections do not apply. To solve this problem, a different set of transfer coefficients required to be derived from the image space of Frank (Edenbrandt, Houston and Macfarlane, 1994). The coefficients can be found in Table 3.3.

Table 3.3 Coefficients for deriving the orthogonal leads X, Y and Z from a paediatric 12-lead ECG. See text for explanation.

	V_{4R}	V_1	V_2	V_4	V_5	V_6	I	II
X	–0.128	–0.122	0.009	0.275	0.251	0.185	0.160	0.013
Y	0.073	0.019	–0.087	–0.065	0.025	0.051	–0.235	0.891
Z	0.072	0.278	0.439	0.189	0.016	–0.084	0.023	–0.128

3.4 The 12-lead vectorcardiogram

3.4.1 Examples of the 12-lead vectorcardiogram

Given that the leads X, Y, Z can be derived from the 12-lead ECG, it follows that the vectorcardiogram can then be derived from the leads X, Y, Z so obtained. This has come to be known as the 12-lead vectorcardiogram. Several studies comparing the derived vectorcardiogram with the original have been undertaken. For example, Edenbrandt and Pahlm (1988) showed that the Inverse Dower method compared more favourably with the original Frank lead vectorcardiogram than did either of two other methods using simple relationships as described in 3.3.2. In a larger study, Kors et al. (1990) compared a regression method and the Inverse Dower method with the Frank lead system itself and found the former to be slightly better from a mathematical stand-point but found no differences between derived vectorcardiograms and the original Frank vectorcardiograms from a clinical point of view, i.e. with respect to the opinion of three blinded reviewers.

Figure 3.3 gives a comparison of three methods of deriving the transverse plane vectorcardiographic QRS loops from the 12-lead ECG and comparing the results with the original Frank lead vectorcardiogram. Considerable variation between methods can be seen.

The remainder of this book will be concerned with examples of the vectorcardiogram derived from the 12-lead ECG using the Inverse Dower method described in 3.3.4 above. Figures 3.4 and 3.5 provide examples of the 12-lead ECG and corresponding vectorcardiograms derived using this method. A similar form of presentation will be used where relevant throughout the book.

There has been no study of the vectorcardiogram derived from the 12-lead ECG in children other than that of Edenbrandt, Houston and Macfarlane (1994). A small comparison of Frank vectorcardiograms versus the 12-lead vectorcardiograms using the new coefficients was undertaken and it was shown that the difference between the two was comparable with day-to-day variation in vectorcardiogram recordings using the Frank system on each occasion (Willems et al., 1972). A comparison of the original Frank vectorcardiogram and the 12-lead vectorcardiogram in an infant is shown in Figure 3.6. Small differences between the two can be seen.

3.4.2 Differences between Frank and 12-lead vectorcardiograms

It is inevitable that the 12-lead and the Frank vectorcardiogram will show differences. It is the authors' contention that this is of limited significance if the normal limits of the 12-lead vectorcardiogram can be obtained using large population samples, which are available

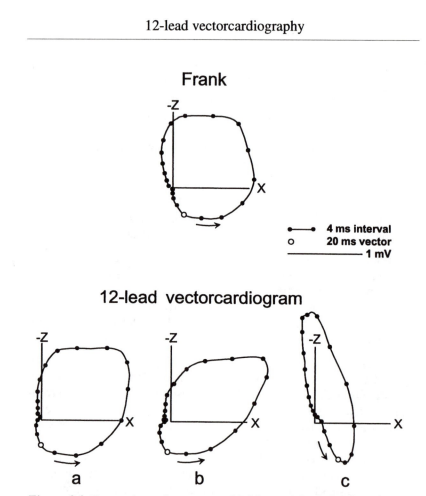

Figure 3.3 *Comparison of transverse QRS loop of the Frank lead vectorcardiogram and three 12-lead QRS vectorcardiographic loops derived in different ways as follows: (a) the inverse Dower method, (b) the method presented by Bjerle and Arvedson, (c) the Marquette method.*

in Glasgow and Lund. The next chapter will discuss the normal ranges of the 12-lead vectorcardiogram, using the Inverse Dower method introduced by Edenbrandt and Pahlm (1988).

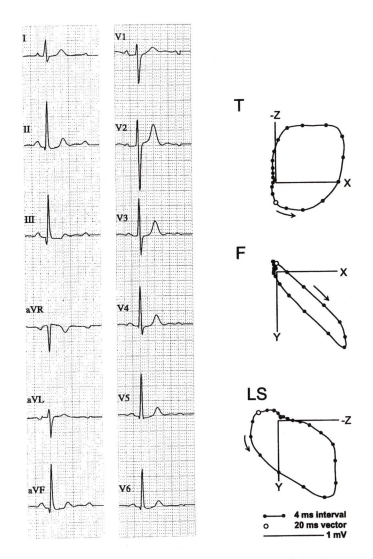

Figure 3.4 *Normal 12-lead ECG and corresponding 12-lead vectorcardiogram, recorded from a 52-year-old female.*

39

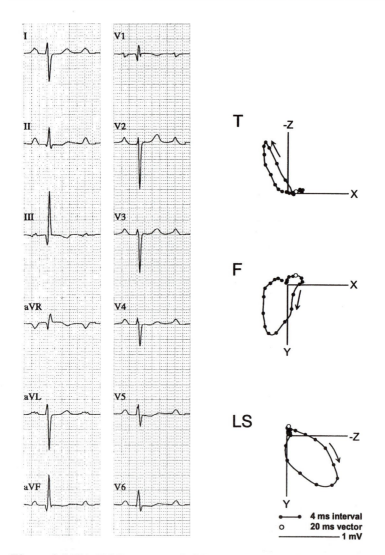

Figure 3.5 *This ECG was recorded from a 30-year-old woman with right ventricular hypertrophy secondary to an atrial septal defect. She also had an anterior myocardial infarction proven clinically and confirmed by radionuclide scintigraphy. She had diabetes mellitus from 1.5 years of age.*

40

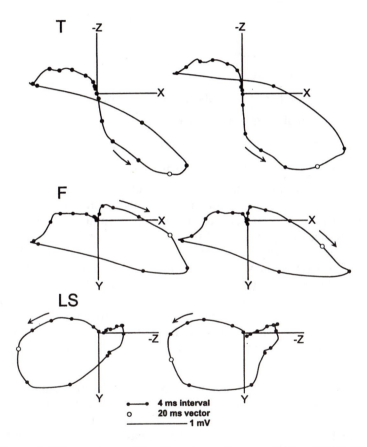

Figure 3.6 Comparison of Frank vectorcardiogram (left) and 12-lead vectorcardiogram (right) in an infant.

4 NORMAL RANGES

4.1 Introduction

The aim of good diagnostic criteria is to separate normal from abnormal with the highest possible sensitivity and specificity. It may be superfluous to repeat well known definitions but for the avoidance of doubt, the following apply:

$$\text{Specificity} = A / B$$

$$\text{Sensitivity} = C / D$$

where   A = number of normals correctly reported as normal

B = total number of normals

C = number of abnormals correctly reported as abnormal

D = total number of abnormals.

Figure 4.1 shows the distribution of Q wave duration in lead Y for normals and for a group of patients with inferior myocardial infarction. If a value of 20 ms is chosen as the upper limit of normal it can be seen that the specificity of the criteria would be approximately 83%. The sensitivity for inferior infarction would be the order of 79%. However, some would argue that 83% specificity, i.e. close to one in five normals reported as abnormal, is not high enough and might adjust the borderline value to 25 ms. In this case, the specificity would increase to 97% and the sensitivity for infarction would decrease to 65%. This process can be continued. For example, with a borderline of 30 ms, specificity is over 99% but sensitivity decreases to 54%.

It is possible to plot the relationship between sensitivity and specificity on what is known as a receiver operating characteristic (ROC) curve. This is shown in Figure 4.2. The point on the curve which approaches closest to 100% sensitivity and specificity, i.e. the top left hand corner, is often regarded as being optimum. In the case of

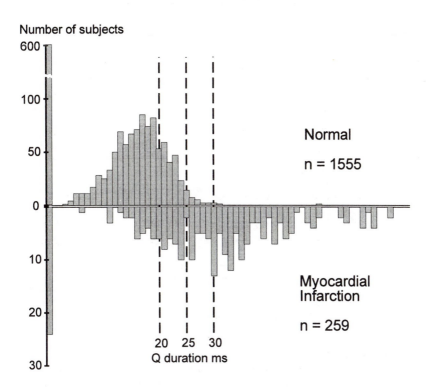

Figure 4.1 *Distribution of Q duration in lead Y in a group of 1555 normal subjects and in a group of 259 patients with inferior myocardial infarction. For explanation, see text.*

electrocardiography, it is often preferable to choose a point on the curve with higher specificity (e.g. 25 ms point in Figure 4.2).

While it is clear that ROC curves are dependent on a knowledge of measurements from a normal population and patients with a particular abnormality, it should also be noted that if a user decides that 95% specificity is the desired level, then knowledge of the abnor-

43

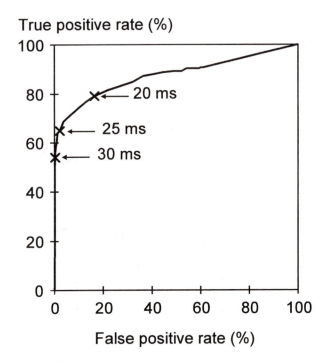

Figure 4.2 *ROC curve showing the relationship between true positive rate (sensitivity) and false positive rate (100 - specificity) for different limits of Q duration in lead Y. The curve is based on the data in Figure 4.1.*

mal data are not required. This is perhaps an extreme view but it emphasises the value of having well defined normal data.

In Glasgow, every effort has been made over the past 10 years to gather a population of controls from birth upwards, in order to meet the objectives outlined above. The remainder of this chapter will deal with the techniques involved and present the results obtained.

4.2 Data acquisition

4.2.1 Techniques

Data have been gathered using two separate types of electrocardiographs each with a common factor of sampling electrocardiographic waveforms at 500 samples/s. All of the recordings made outside Glasgow Royal Infirmary, e.g. on infants and children, were gathered using a Mingorec 4 from Siemens-Elema AB, Solna, Sweden. This acquires eight leads simultaneously, converts from analogue to digital form at a rate of 500 samples/s and writes the output to a digital cassette tape, which is then replayed on a computer from Digital Equipment Corporation (DEC) for further analysis.

For ECGs recorded within Glasgow Royal Infirmary, an electrocardiograph designed and constructed within the Department of Medical Cardiology was used (Watts and Shoat, 1987). This device was connected by a broadband network from wards and clinics to the central DEC computing facility within the Department.

The methods for analysing the ECGs have been described in detail elsewhere (Macfarlane et al., 1990a) but are summarised very briefly here.

Up to 8 seconds of ECG with all leads sampled simultaneously, are processed initially to remove baseline wander, if present, and also any AC interference. Thereafter, QRS detection is undertaken. The same methods apply whether the ECG is recorded from a neonate or an adult. The QRS complexes so detected are then typed into different morphologies and logic selects one particular morphology for analysis. All PQRST cycles of that morphology are then averaged to form a single synthesized beat (with all 12 leads effectively recorded simultaneously). The derived leads X, Y, Z are then obtained using the equations of 3.3.4. The wave measurement program then locates the onsets and terminations of the various P, QRS and T components in order to measure amplitudes and durations.

Rhythm analysis is then undertaken. This uses some measurements from the average beat matrix but also three complete leads from the initial recording. Generally these would be II, III and V_1. When rhythm has been determined, diagnostic logic is then entered to interpret the measurements from the average beats. Several hundred diagnostic statements can be output by the program. The same program can now be used for adults as well as for children (Macfarlane et al., 1990b). In other words, the ability to interpret ECGs from children is not an optional add-on to the logic but is integral to the diagnostic criteria. Some details are presented elsewhere (Macfarlane et al., 1989b).

4.2.2 Sampling methods

Different approaches to the selection of an apparently healthy population can be adopted. For example, age and sex registers can be used (Lundh, 1984) but the technique adopted for adults in the Glasgow data was essentially to seek volunteers from different departments of local government, e.g. teaching, administration, building etc. All individuals admitted to the normal group were seen by a physician who obtained a complete history and undertook a physical examination. The usual blood tests were performed and in the initial part of the study, chest X-rays were obtained. It was found that a positive yield from chest X-rays was essentially nil and latterly they were discontinued as part of the screening procedure.

For sampling from children, the procedure was different. Recordings were obtained from a maternity hospital with the full consent of parents. In the pre-school children, it was necessary to visit postnatal clinics, health centres and playgroups in order to obtain recordings from children, again with permission of parents. Recordings were obtained from school children by installing the Siemens electrocardiograph for periods in different schools with the permission of the local health and education authority. Volunteers were sought subject to parental permission.

4.2.3 Population data

1,555 adults were entered into the normal database. The age and sex distribution is shown in Figure 4.3. There tends to be a preponderance of males over 30 years of age, probably because of the predominance of male workers of that age group.

Figure 4.4 shows similar data for 1,782 healthy neonates, infants and children from whom ECGs were recorded. It should be pointed out that in this age group, lead V_{4R} was used in preference to lead V_3 as is the custom in many countries.

Actual numbers of males and females in the total group of 3,337 are given in Table 4.1.

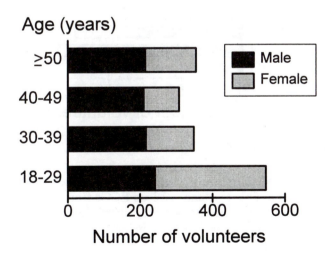

Figure 4.3 *Age/sex distribution of the normal adult database. Further details are provided in Table 4.1.*

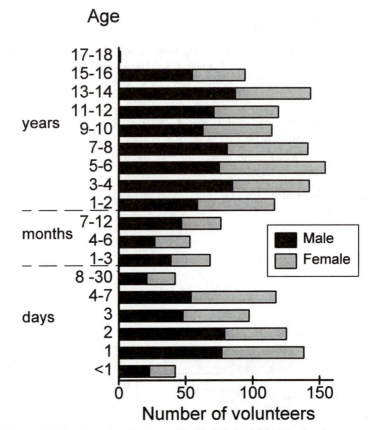

Figure 4.4 *Age/sex distribution of the normal children's database. Further details are provided in Table 4.1.*

In Taiwan, in collaboration with the Veterans' General Hospital in Taipei, it was possible to obtain 12-lead ECGs from 503 apparently healthy Chinese individuals (Chen et al., 1989). From these, the 12-lead vectorcardiogram has been obtained (Yang et al., 1993). Essentially, methods used were similar to those for the collection of adult data in Caucasians although a higher percentage of individuals was in hospital with non-cardiac problems.

Table 4.1 Numbers of males and females in the total population group.

Age	Male	Female	Total
≤ 24 hours	23	19	
1 day	77	61	
2	79	46	
3	48	49	
4–7	54	63	
≤ 1 month	21	21	
≤ 3	39	29	
≤ 6	27	26	
≤ 1 year	47	29	
1–2 years	59	57	
3–4	85	57	
5–6	75	79	
7–8	81	60	
9–10	63	51	
11–12	71	48	
13–14	87	56	
15–16	55	39	
17–18	0	1	
Children Σ	991	791	1782
18–29	242	304	
30–39	217	131	
40–49	210	97	
≥ 50	215	139	
Adult Σ	884	671	1555
Total Σ			3337

4.2.4 Methods of analysis

All measurements from each recording were stored on computer file and added to a database. The adult and paediatric data were kept separate.

The BMDP suite of statistical programs was available for obtaining the basic data such as mean and standard deviation etc. The programs mainly used were P2D and P6D.

4.2.5 Statistical considerations

It has been known for many years that in general terms, ECG data are not normally distributed but tend to be skewed. An illustration is shown in Figure 4.5. For this reason, normal ranges are best described not by using the mean $\pm$ twice the standard deviation but by 96 percentile ranges, i.e. by excluding 2% of measurements at the top and bottom end of a particular set of measurements. Wherever possible this has been done in analysing the data. Only in the case of small numbers such as, for example, healthy males with a Q wave in V_1, was it necessary to include the complete range because total numbers were too small. One other point that should be noted is that the calculation of the mean is based only on measurements which were present. In other words, if there were 100 patients in a particular group but only 40 had an S wave in a selected lead, then the mean amplitude was derived using only the 40 measurements and the 60 values of 0 mV for the remaining patients were excluded from the calculation of the mean.

With respect to angular data, care was taken to ensure that all measurements were in a meaningful range. In other words, the recommendations for measuring angles would suggest that the direction in the frontal plane of the X axis would be labelled as $0°$. If a vector measurement inferior to that was perhaps $20°$ and one superior to the X axis was $340°$, the mean value would certainly not be $180°$ but $0°$. In other words, $340°$ would be converted to $-20°$ before calculating the mean value. Alternative methods for dealing with angular data were elaborated many years ago by Downs et al. (1965).

4.3 Results - scalar data

4.3.1 Wave amplitudes and durations

The relevant tables of normal limits of PQRST amplitudes and durations in the derived leads X, Y and Z are presented in Appendix 1. Again, it can be confirmed that effects of age and sex on the amplitudes of waveforms are significant. This can be seen in Figure 4.6 where the mean S wave amplitude in lead Z is presented.

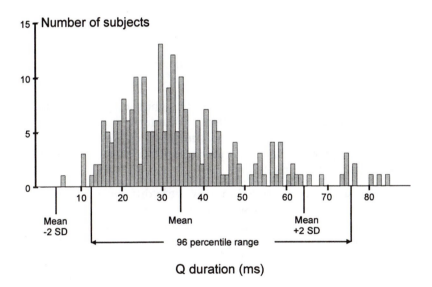

Figure 4.5 *An example of a skewed distribution where there is a long tail of measurements at the upper end of the distribution. The figure shows a histogram of Q wave duration in lead Y in a group of 259 patients with proven inferior myocardial infarction. 24 patients with no Q waves in lead Y are excluded from the calculation of the mean.*

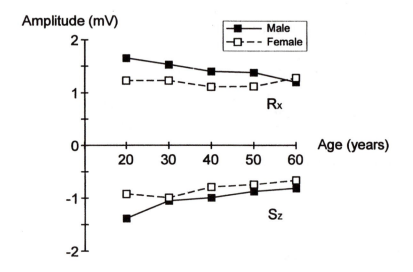

Figure 4.6 *Effect of age and sex on mean R wave amplitude in lead X and mean S wave amplitude in lead Z.*

Here the amplitude in young males is significantly higher than in young females, although the difference diminishes as age increases. These findings are similar to measurements of the S wave in V_2. The effect is not so marked for the mean R wave in lead X which is also shown in the same figure.

In contrast, durations tended to show little difference between different age and sex groups with the exception of the QRS duration which, as is well known, is approximately 8 ms longer in males than in females although strangely almost no cognisance is taken of this in any diagnostic criteria.

4.3.2 Paediatric data

It goes without saying that dramatic changes in paediatric measurements can be seen from birth onwards. Again, appropriate tables are presented in Appendix 2. As an example, the upper limit of normal S wave amplitude in lead X is shown in Figure 4.7. There is a rapid

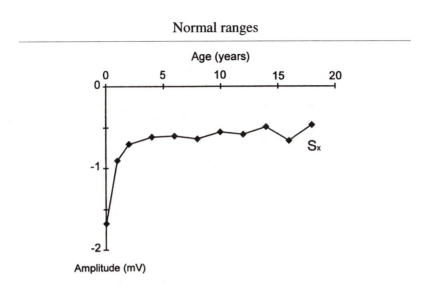

Figure 4.7 *The upper limit of normal S_X amplitude in children from birth to adolescence.*

decrease in S_X amplitude in the first year of life corresponding to a counter-clockwise shift of the maximum frontal plane QRS vector.

4.3.3 Comparative vectorcardiography

Yang and Macfarlane (1994) recently reported on a comparison of the 12-lead vectorcardiogram in apparently healthy Caucasians and Chinese. 503 Chinese were added to the database of 1,555 Caucasians giving a total of 2,058 individuals whose vectorcardiograms were derived from the conventional 12-lead ECG.

The trend of the influence of age and sex on the magnitude and direction of the derived QRS and T vectors was found to be similar in both cases. In the younger age groups, the magnitude of the maximal spatial vector was essentially greater in Caucasians than in Chinese while in the older age groups over 40, the reverse was the case. This was a somewhat surprising finding for which there is no clear explanation. Figures 4.8 and 4.9 show a comparison between the QRS and T vector magnitude in both races. It can be seen that it is essential to include the effect of age, sex and race when interpreting 12-lead vectorcardiographic appearances.

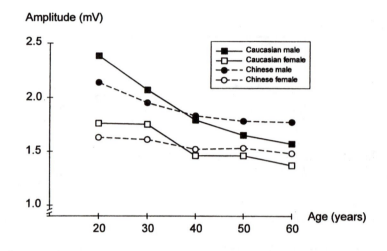

Figure 4.8 *Mean magnitude of the maximal QRS vector amplitude in Caucasians and Chinese.*

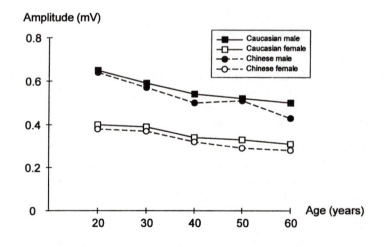

Figure 4.9 *Mean magnitude of the maximal T vector amplitude in Caucasians and Chinese.*

4.4 Results - vector data

4.4.1 P loops

In the infant, the P loop tends to be directed vertically at birth but it soon rotates superiorly in the frontal plane and remains around 55°. In the transverse plane, the P loop in children at birth is approximately 20° to 25° and subsequently shifts a little towards the adult value of around 0°. Sex differences between the mean P wave vector in the transverse plane are significant with the mean direction for males being 349° and for females 14° (Draper et al., 1964, Nemati et al., 1978). It should be noted that the results obtained by these authors were derived using the Frank system.

4.4.2 QRS loops

There is, of course, a considerable change from birth to adulthood in the QRS loop in the 12-lead vectocardiogram. Figure 4.10 shows a 12-lead QRS loop from a neonate where the maximum QRS vector is oriented around 150° in the frontal plane. On the other hand, in the normal adult QRS in the frontal plane, Figure 4.11, the QRS loop is oriented at around 50°. In general terms, in the frontal plane the QRS loop is in the vast majority of cases inscribed in a clockwise direction in the infant. In the adult, the frontal plane loop can be inscribed either in a clockwise or counter clockwise direction although again, the clockwise loop tends to predominate. In the transverse plane, in the neonate, the inscription around birth is 43% clockwise and 45% counterclockwise but soon changes to being almost totally counter clockwise as it is in the normal adult. A figure-of-eight loop can be found in 20 to 40% of children up to 8 months of age using the Frank system (Namin et al., 1964) although our own 12-lead data suggest a lower incidence. Table 4.2 shows the results derived from the Glasgow data in respect of direction of inscription of the QRS loops in the frontal and transverse planes.

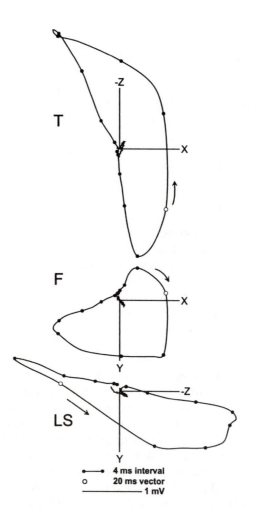

Figure 4.10 12-lead QRS and T loops from a healthy neonate.

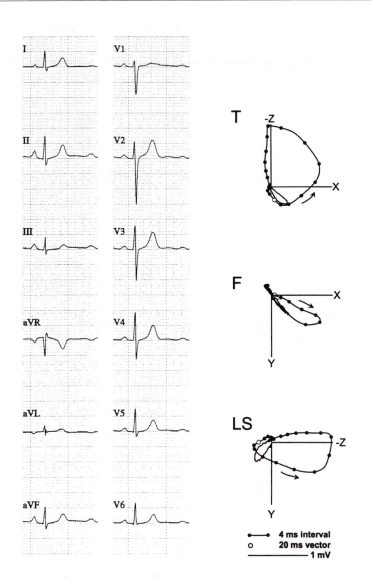

Figure 4.11 *12-lead QRS and T loops from a healthy adult.*

Table 4.2 Direction of inscription of the QRS vector loop in transverse and frontal planes expressed as a percentage from 1,555 adult Caucasian normals. (CCW; Counterclockwise Rotation, CW; Clockwise Rotation)

Planes		CCW	Figure of 8	CW
Transverse	Male	98.1	0.9	1.0
	Female	97.9	1.2	0.9
Frontal	Male	22.9	19.1	58.0
	Female	21.8	25.3	52.9

4.4.3 Left axis deviation

It may seem superfluous to consider a discussion on left axis deviation but the normal range of the maximum QRS vector in the frontal plane is, indeed, quite different in the 12-lead vectorcardiogram from that in the standard 12-lead ECG. A full list of ranges is given in the Appendix.

It can be seen that in healthy females, for example, the maximum QRS vector is never superior to 0°. In males, this seems to occur in a few individuals in the 30–59 years age group but, by and large, the vast majority of individuals have a maximum QRS vector inferior to 0°. This suggests the following criteria:

Borderline left axis deviation: $0^{\circ} \rightarrow -15^{\circ}$

Left axis deviation: $-15^{\circ} \rightarrow -90^{\circ}$

4.4.4 Right axis deviation

The tables in the Appendix indicate that with the exception of young males < 30 years of age, the normal maximum QRS vector in the frontal plane is always $< 65^{\circ}$. This is considerably different from the normal frontal plane vector derived from the 12-lead ECG. It does suggest that the following criteria be used:

Borderline right axis deviation:

Females and (males > 30 years)	$65° \rightarrow 75°$
Males < 30 years	$90° \rightarrow 100°$

Right axis deviation:

Females and (males > 30 years)	$> 75°$
Males < 30 years	$> 100°$

4.4.5 T loops

From Figures 4.10 and 4.11 discussed above, the direction of the maximum T vector in the frontal and transverse planes can be seen for the average newborn and the average adult. It follows that there is a gradual change of T vector orientation from one position to another with increasing age. Details of some T vector measurements can be found in the Appendices.

5 HYPERTROPHY

5.1 Introduction

5.1.1 What is hypertrophy?

Electrocardiographers tend to report the pattern of increased voltage in the lateral leads together with accompanying STT changes as left ventricular hypertrophy (LVH). The advent of echocardiography as well as cardiac catheterisation has meant that the variety of pathologies which constitute the generic term 'hypertrophy' is now better known. In general terms, hypertrophy can be taken to mean an increase in mass. All four chambers of the heart can demonstrate hypertrophy or enlargement either in isolation or in combination. Enlargement is a term that is perhaps more associated with an increase in volume whereas hypertrophy strictly may relate to an increase in muscle mass.

The sub-division of different types of hypertrophy is essentially based around left ventricular geometry. Where there is an overall increase in mass with a dominant increase in muscle thickness without an increase in cavity volume, the term concentric hypertrophy is used. Where there is an increase in mass predominantly due to an increase in volume, the term eccentric hypertrophy is used.

Huwez, Pringle and Macfarlane (1992) have recently introduced a new classification for hypertrophy on the basis of mass and volume. The different types and the criteria are given in Table 5.1. A salutary lesson from that study was that a patient with apparently normal mass and volume could demonstrate the ECG changes of LVH described above. In addition, both concentric and eccentric hypertrophy could produce similar ECG changes or none at all.

Notwithstanding the above, the remainder of this chapter is generally concerned with the classical description of vectorcardiographic changes accompanying hypertrophy.

Table 5.1 Left ventricular geometry classification.

Left ventricular		Type
mass	volume	
normal	normal	normal
normal	increased	isolated left ventricular volume overload
increased	normal	concentric LVH
increased	increased	eccentric LVH

5.1.2 Effects of age, sex and race

It will be apparent from the previous chapter on normal ranges, that QRS voltage in some leads such as X and Z increases with age until early adulthood and then decreases again. Likewise, it has also been shown that, in many cases, sex differences particularly with respect to voltage can be demonstrated in vectorcardiographic parameters. Similar effects can be seen within different races.

All of this suggests that criteria for ventricular hypertrophy have to be based on a knowledge of all of these three variables.

5.1.3 Value of vectorcardiography

It goes without saying that the echocardiogram gives a detailed picture of left ventricular geometry. On the other hand, it is the ECG that may demonstrate secondary STT changes which are well known to be associated with a poor prognosis (Kannell, 1983; Macfarlane, 1987). If a reasonable specificity of 95% is desired, then the best ECG criteria have a sensitivity around 50%. Data such as these vary from one study to another depending on the gold standard which may be post-mortem weights on the one hand or echocardiographic measurements on the other. The reader should therefore be aware, from the outset, that the vectorcardiographic diagnosis of LVH is somewhat insensitive.

5.2 Atrial enlargement

In the normal 12-lead vectorcardiogram, the P wave may exhibit two distinct components which probably result from asynchronous depolarisation of the left and right atrium. In this event, the bifid nature of the P wave is best seen in the inferior lead Y. In view of the fact that normal atrial depolarisation commences in the right atrium before spreading to the left atrium, it follows that the first component is due to right atrial excitation and the second to left atrial excitation.

5.2.1 Right atrial enlargement

One of the manifestations of right atrial enlargement is a P wave in the inferior lead Y with an amplitude > 0.3 mV. As this abnormality not infrequently occurs in respiratory disorders, it is sometimes called P pulmonale (Figure 5.1). Occasionally, P_Y may be of normal amplitude but there may be a prominent P_Z > 0.15 mV on account of right atrial enlargement.

Chou and Helm (1965) have pointed out that P wave changes in the inferior lead Y occasionally resemble P pulmonale when there are no clinical findings to support such a diagnosis. The cause of the abnormal P wave may be left atrial hypertrophy and the term 'pseudo P pulmonale' is used to describe such a phenomenon. Clearly, this diagnosis should be made on the basis of the clinical findings taken in conjunction with the ECG appearances.The normal ranges of the projections of the maximum P vector on to the three planes are so wide that little diagnostic advantage can be gained from a study of these parameters in respect of right atrial enlargement.

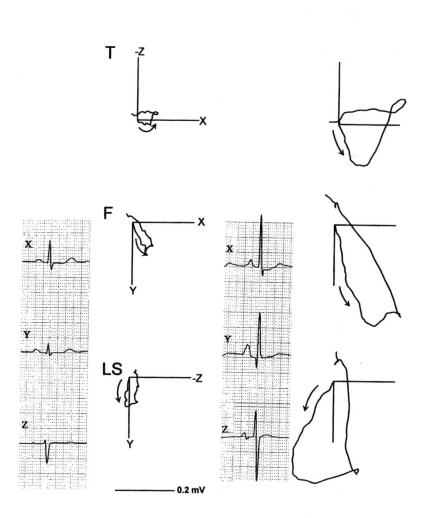

Figure 5.1 *Normal P loops (left) and an example of combined atrial enlargement (right).*

5.2.2 Left atrial enlargement

When left atrial enlargement occurs, several abnormalities may result. Firstly, the P wave duration may be increased beyond 120 ms. Secondly, bifid or M shaped P waves of greater than normal duration may be found in the inferior lead Y and this pattern is often referred to as P mitrale because of its common association with mitral stenosis. From the vectorcardiographic point of view, enlargement of the left atrium may also cause an increase in the left atrial vectors which in turn produce a rotation of the terminal portion of the P wave vector posteriorly and to the left (Figure 5.1). Thus, the terminal component of the scalar P wave in lead Z can be increased in negativity and in duration.

The maximum P vector amplitude may be increased but the normal range of P vector orientation is so wide as to be of little value. On occasions, the maximum P vector magnitude may exceed 0.3 mV when the individual scalar components are within normal. In this case, left atrial enlargement is the most likely cause.

5.2.3 Combined atrial enlargement

In general terms, a combination of the individual criteria for left and right atrial enlargement when present would be suggestive of combined atrial enlargement (Figure 5.1).

5.3 Left ventricular hypertrophy

5.3.1 Diagnostic criteria

When LVH or left ventricular enlargement produces alterations in QRS morphology, these relate generally to an increase in QRS vector amplitude. On occasions, the maximum QRS vector will be rotated posteriorly and this is seen best in the transverse plane where the resultant effect is to produce an increase in the amplitude of S_Z. Consideration of the basic principles of vectorcardiography indicates that if a vectorcardiographic loop rotates posteriorly increasing S_Z, then R_X would decrease simultaneously. Thus, one of the commonly used vectorcardiographic criteria is based on $R_X + S_Z$. The data from the 1,555 patients in the Glasgow database suggest that the upper limit of $R_X + S_Z = 3.95$ mV for males over 40 years of age. It is, however, possible to express the upper limit of normal for males as a continuous age dependent equation as follows:

$$R_X + S_Z = [72.81 - 0.02074 \text{ age(months)}]^2 \, \mu V$$

Similar equations apply for women and for Chinese.

The typical vectorcardiographic appearances in LVH are shown in Figure 5.2. In this case, there is increased magnitude of the QRS vector which is more posteriorly oriented than the mean maximum QRS vector in normals in the transverse plane while the T loop is oppositely directed to the QRS loop. This is equivalent to the secondary STT pattern in the lateral leads.

It should be noted that the individual component amplitudes of the scalar leads may be normal while the resultant vector amplitude can be abnormal. For example, if the amplitude of R_X is 2.4 mV and, at the same instant, R_Y is 1.5 mV and S_Z is 1.5 mV (although corresponding peak amplitudes might be a little higher), it follows that the amplitude of the maximum QRS vector would be

$$3.2\text{mV} = \sqrt{(2.4^2 + 1.5^2 + 1.5^2)} \text{ mV}$$

Each of the scalar amplitudes is within normal range for a male aged 45 but the vector magnitude is outside normal (see Appendix 1).

Various types of QRS loop may be seen in the vectorcardiogram. These are best differentiated by appearances in the transverse plane. Type I may simply resemble a normal QRS loop but be of increased magnitude. In Type II, there is a rotation of the projection of the maximum QRS vector posteriorly beyond 310° in the transverse

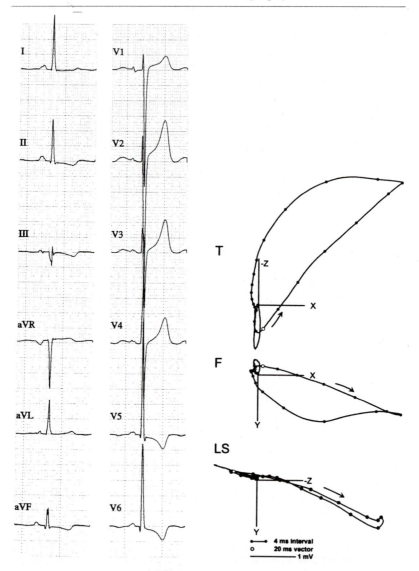

Figure 5.2 *An example of LVH Type I. Note the increased magnitude of the QRS loops best seen in the transverse plane where the T loop is essentially oppositely directed to the QRS loop.*

plane (Figure 5.3), possibly with a normal QRS voltage. It is not common, however, to find an abnormal orientation of the QRS vector loop in LVH without voltage evidence in addition. In Type III where LVH is very marked, there may be a figure of eight loop in the transverse plane with the distal part of the loop inscribed in a clockwise direction (Figure 5.4). In Type IV, there may be slightly increased QRS duration, and an abnormally large QRS maximum vector, but the rate of inscription of the loop is slower than normal as manifested by the closeness of the dots. This pattern is sometimes called 'incomplete left bundle branch block (LBBB)' which often accompanies LVH.

Reference has already been made to secondary STT changes (Figure 5.2) sometimes called left ventricular strain or overload pattern. In a series of patients (Huwez, 1990), it was found that this pattern of ST depression with assymetric T wave inversion was 94% sensitive for LVH. Thus, even in the absence of high voltage, this ECG finding in the scalar lead X should be regarded as a pointer towards the diagnosis of LVH.

One further point can be made concerning the vectorcardiographic appearances in severe LVH. It can happen that the initial QRS vectors are directed posteriorly, i.e. there is a Q wave in the anteroseptal lead Z or V_2. This makes the differential diagnosis of anteroseptal infarction from LVH difficult unless the clinical picture is relatively clear cut. For example, Figure 5.5 shows such a pattern in a 73-year-old male with hypertension and aortic stenosis and insufficiency. The reasons for the presence of the Q wave are not fully understood although many hypotheses have been put forward. Possibly on account of there being three areas of initial activation in the left ventricle, the concept of the genesis of the Q wave may be revised. It could be postulated that the electrical activation of the area of the left ventricle adjacent to the posterior wall which is among the first to be depolarised, predominates on account of left ventricular wall thickness, thereby leading to initial QRS forces oriented posteriorly producing a Q wave in the anteroseptal lead.

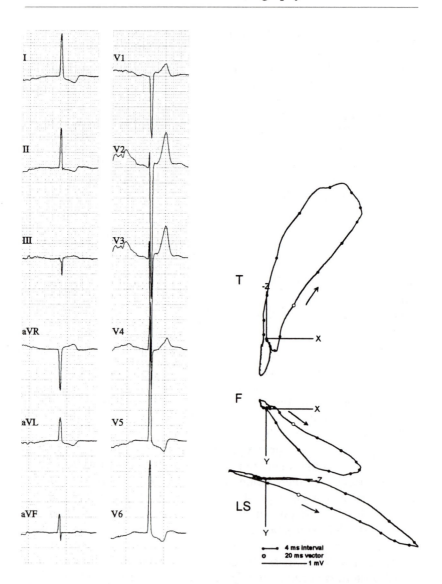

Figure 5.3 *An example of LVH Type II. Note that the maximum QRS vector in the transverse plane is posterior to 300°.*

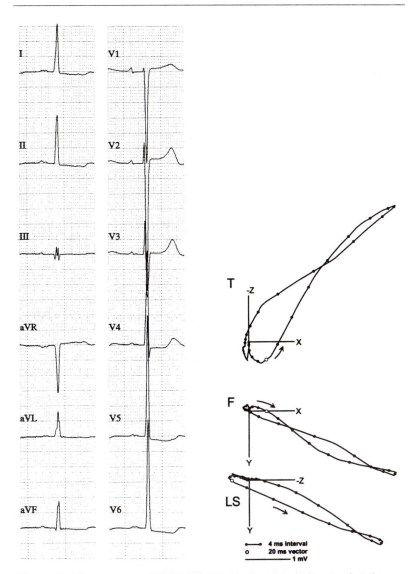

Figure 5.4 *An example of LVH Type III. In this case, a figure-of-eight loop can be seen clearly in the transverse plane while the maximum QRS vector exceeds 4 mV.*

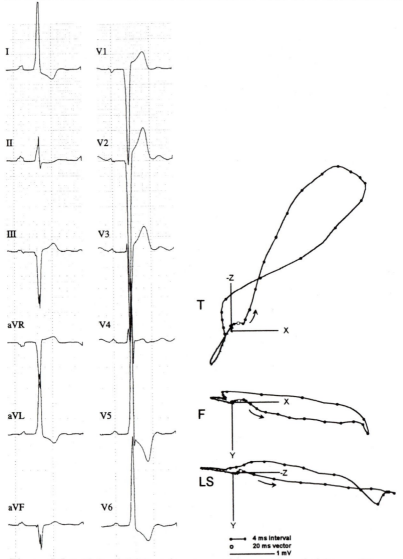

Figure 5.5 *A 12-lead ECG and vectorcardiogram recorded from a 73-year-old male with hypertension and aortic stenosis and insufficiency. Note that the initial QRS vectors are directed posteriorly, i.e. there is a Q wave in lead Z. Other typical features of LVH can also be seen.*

Other criteria which point to LVH include left axis deviation which, in the vectorcardiogram, is a QRS axis superior to $0°$ in the frontal plane. Indeed, apart from the specific criteria of increased vector magnitude and posteriorly rotated maximum QRS vector orientation, other criteria mirror those for the conventional 12-lead ECG, e.g. a delayed intrinsicoid deflection in lead X and increased P terminal force in lead Z.

5.3.2 Bundle branch block and LVH

The diagnosis of LVH from an ECG which shows bundle branch block is controversial. Some authors have claimed it is possible to make such a diagnosis while others have noted in various series that in the presence of LBBB, LVH is always found. Thus, no specific criteria for the diagnosis of LVH and LBBB are presented here. However, one or two points can be made.

As will be seen in Chapter 7, the vectorcardiographic appearances in LBBB are characteristic in having a narrow QRS loop in the transverse plane. If the scalar lead appears to have the LBBB pattern with a tall R_X but does not have the narrow bundle branch block loop, then LVH could be considered as a possible cause (incomplete LBBB/LVH pattern).

5.4 Right ventricular hypertrophy

Increased right ventricular excitation forces or increased right ventricular volume can produce varying ECG patterns depending on the time of the occurrence of the abnormal electrical activity compared to that of the left ventricle. Hypertrophy of the free wall of the right ventricle will produce abnormal anterior forces in early ventricular depolarisation whereas basal hypertrophy will produce abnormal posterior forces late in ventricular depolarisation. In the vectorcardiogram, there are essentially two presentations of right ventricular hypertrophy (RVH), namely, a prominent R wave in lead Z and a deep S wave in lead X. The presence of these abnormalities either singly or together produces four patterns of RVH or enlargement. These are as follows:

5.4.1 RVH - Type A

Type A RVH is manifested as an increase in the ratio of anterior/posterior forces in the transverse plane with counterclockwise inscription of the QRS loop (Figure 5.6). Often the abnormal QRS loop may have a T loop directed posteriorly corresponding to the secondary ST-T abnormalities sometimes seen in V_1 and V_2.

One criterion of value in Type A is the projection of the maximum QRS vector onto the transverse plane $> 30^0$. Occasionally, this may be present when voltage and ratio measurements in the anteroseptal leads are normal.

5.4.2 RVH - Type B

One of the major advantages of the vectorcardiogram is preservation of the timing relationships between the different scalar leads. Thus, while two different scalar patterns may have similar appearances, the vectorcardiogram can be normal in one and abnormal in another. This is often apparent in Type B RVH. In this case, the QRS loop in the transverse plane initially has normal counterclockwise inscription but the second part of the loop is deviated anteriorly so that the net effect is to have a loop with clockwise or figure of eight inscription in the transverse plane (Figure 5.7).

5.4.3 RVH - Type C

The third type of RVH is manifested as an abnormal transverse plane vectorcardiographic loop that is normally counter-clockwise inscribed with the maximum QRS vector being oriented posteriorly and to the right (Figure 5.8). This pattern is most often found in patients with chronic respiratory disease and therefore may be accompanied by P pulmonale. However, some patients with mitral stenosis also exhibit such findings. It is thought that the posterior

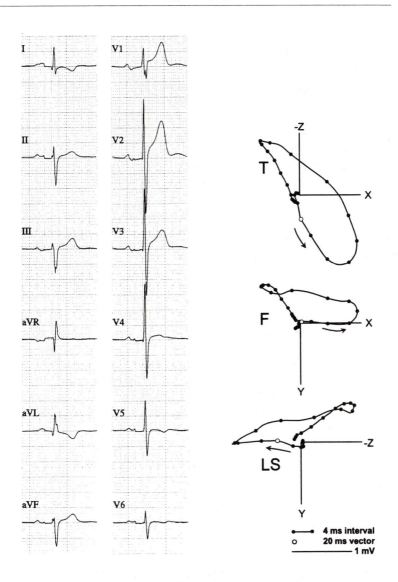

Figure 5.6 *An example of RVH Type A where there is a marked increase in anteriorly directed forces as seen in the transverse plane.*

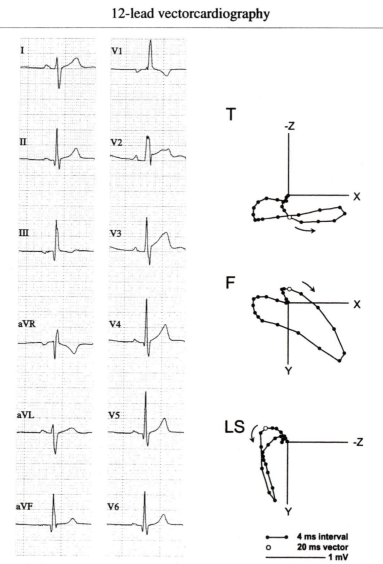

Figure 5.7 *An example of RVH Type B where there is a figure-of-eight loop in the transverse plane in which all forces are seen to be anteriorly oriented. Note the late rightward directed forces corresponding to the deep S wave in lead I.*

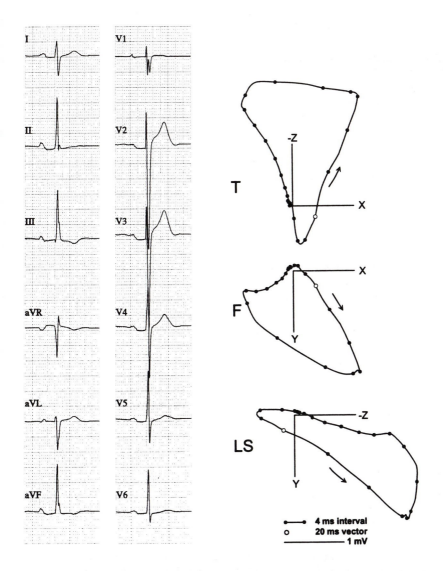

Figure 5.8 *An example of RVH Type C. In this case, there is a large posterior and rightward directed force in the later part of QRS.*

75

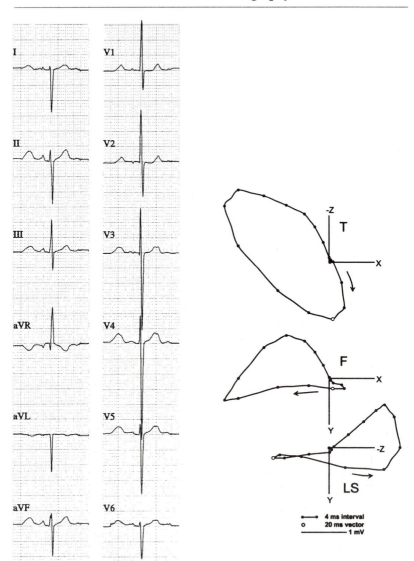

Figure 5.9 *An example of RVH Type D where the QRS loop in the transverse plane is clearly abnormal, being inscribed in a clockwise direction and lying almost entirely to the right. Marked right axis deviation can also be seen in the frontal plane loop.*

rightward displacement of the QRS vector is due to hypertrophy of the basal portion of the right ventricle. Secondary STT changes can also be found in this pattern. The abnormal rightward forces also translate into right axis deviation in the frontal plane.

5.4.4 RVH - Type D

In the more severe forms of RVH, as may occur in certain forms of congenital heart disease the main QRS vector may be directed abnormally not only to the anterior but also to the right with clockwise inscription of QRS in the transverse plane (Figure 5.9).

5.5 Combined ventricular hypertrophy

It has been claimed that in most cases of LVH there is an accompanying RVH (Gottdiener et al., 1985). The vectorcardiographic diagnosis of biventricular hypertrophy is mainly based on finding features of both LVH and RVH separately. For example, if the transverse QRS loop is directed posteriorly and has an increased magnitude with the T loop oppositely directed, as in secondary changes of LVH, and the frontal QRS vector is oriented around $90°$, then combined ventricular hypertrophy should be considered.

5.6 Paediatric vectorcardiography

The various forms of congenital heart disease can produce a variety of vectorcardiographic patterns which can be extremely difficult to interpret. A few patterns are pathognomonic of rare forms of congenital heart disease but in any event, the report must remain an ECG interpretation. In other words, no attempt should be made to infer the anatomy of the congenital lesion in the majority of cases. Brohet (1990) has reviewed the advantages of vectorcardiography in congenital heart disease.

6 MYOCARDIAL INFARCTION

6.1 Introduction

6.1.1 Theoretical considerations

A myocardial infarction is death of myocardial tissue as a result of insufficient blood supply, i.e. due to a stenosis or occlusion of a coronary artery. An infarcted area is electrically inert and distorts the normal spread of excitation. The net effect is that the electrical forces, which are influenced by the 'dead zone' or infarct vector, are directed away from the area of myocardial infarction. This is in contrast with hypertrophy which produces electrical forces directed towards the area of increased ventricular mass.

6.1.2 Anatomical definitions

There is a lack of unanimity in describing myocardial infarction. In 1978, the American College of Cardiology Conference on Optimal Electrocardiography described myocardial infarction in terms of Q waves seen in the various leads of the 12-lead ECG. This has resulted in terms such as septal, anteroseptal and anterior infarction being used. However, there is still no consensus regarding the localization of an infarction among electrocardiographers.

Radiological or echocardiographic techniques can also be used to detect and localize a myocardial infarction. In coronary angiography, it is not the infarcted area per se which is detected but the stenosis or occlusion of the coronary artery which caused the myocardial infarction. An infarcted area causes abnormalities in the ventricular contraction pattern, which can usually be detected in a left ventriculogram or in an echocardiogram.

The techniques described above show different aspects of the same disease. Differences in the position and orientation of the heart and a variation in the anatomy of the coronary arteries have varying

78

influence on these techniques. Therefore, the correlations between electrocardiographic changes, abnormalities of ventricular contraction and the degree of stenosis in relevant coronary arteries are not excellent. This should be borne in mind when comparing different techniques for the diagnosis of myocardial infarction.

Notwithstanding any of the above, in very general terms, occlusion of a left anterior descending coronary artery or a left main stem artery is likely to produce an infarct predominantly in the anterior (anteroseptal/anterosuperior) wall of the heart. An occlusion in the right coronary artery will generally produce an inferior myocardial infarction while occlusion of the left cirumflex produces a lateral or posterolateral/inferior myocardial infarction.

6.2 The 12-lead vectorcardiogram in myocardial infarction

6.2.1 Anterior infarction

In keeping with the concept of the dead zone or infarct vector, an anterior myocardial infarction will result in slightly increased posteriorly directed electromotive forces and a reduction, if not an absence, of anteriorly directed forces in the early part of ventricular depolarisation. In 12-lead ECG terminology, this corresponds to a QS complex in V_2. The corresponding vectorcardiographic appearances are shown in Figure 6.1. Here it can be seen that there is no electrical activity in the left anterior quadrant of the transverse plane vectorcardiogram. This type of clear-cut myocardial infarction, from an electrocardiographic point-of-view, is generally well delineated on the 12-lead ECG. Of more interest is the situation where the 12-lead ECG may be somewhat equivocal with low R waves in the anterior leads but the vectorcardiogram shows other features which are suggestive of myocardial infarction. In the transverse plane, common vectorcardiographic criteria for anterior myocardial infarction are listed in Table 6.1.

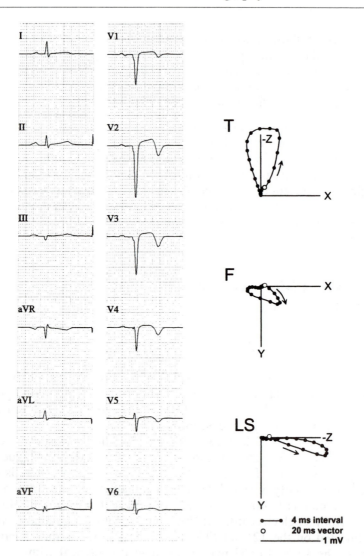

Figure 6.1 *The classical features of anterior myocardial infarction with a complete absence of anteriorly directed QRS vectors. Note that the 30 ms vector is also posterior to 300° in the transverse plane.*

Table 6.1 Criteria for anterior myocardial infarction.

Any of the following in the transverse QRS loop:
direction of 30 ms vector 225° - 300°
loop area in left anterior quadrant < 1% of the total loop area
an early bite, i.e. a clockwise inscription of the loop, with an amplitude > 0.05 mV (see 6.2.8)

Figure 6.2 gives an example of a QRS loop where there are initial anteriorly directed forces but the 30 ms QRS vector is posterior to 300°. Figure 6.3 shows a different form of vectorcardiographic change where there is an initial counter-clockwise inscription leading to a bite in the vectorcardiographic loop (see 6.2.8). Figure 6.4 illustrates a case of anterior myocardial infarction where the area of the QRS loop in the left anterior quadrant < 1%.

6.2.2 Anterior myocardial infarction versus LVH

In cases of severe LVH, the vectorcardiographic loop may also resemble anterior myocardial infarction. In many cases, the difference between the two can clearly be separated on non-electrocardiographic considerations, clearly including the clinical history. If the QRS loop and T loop are oppositely directed in the transverse plane with lack of QRS electrical activity anteriorly, the higher probability is that appearances are due to LVH (Figure 5.5).

Of course, both abnormalities can be present simultaneously in an individual and this is more likely to be the case if the QRS -T angle is approximately 90°. A T vector directed posteriorly to the right suggests an ischaemic component to the abnormality as isolated LVH would rarely produce a T vector so oriented.

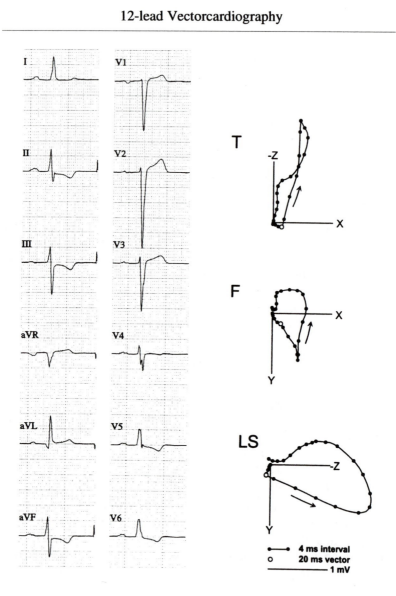

Figure 6.2 *An example of anterior myocardial infarction where the initial QRS forces are anteriorly directed for a little over 20 ms but where the 30 ms vector is just posterior to 300°.*

82

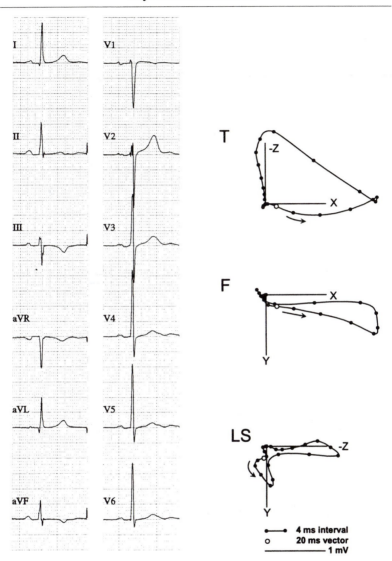

Figure 6.3 *Anterior myocardial infarction proven by diagnostic cardiac catheterization in a 62-year-old male. Note the early bite in the QRS loop in the transverse plane.*

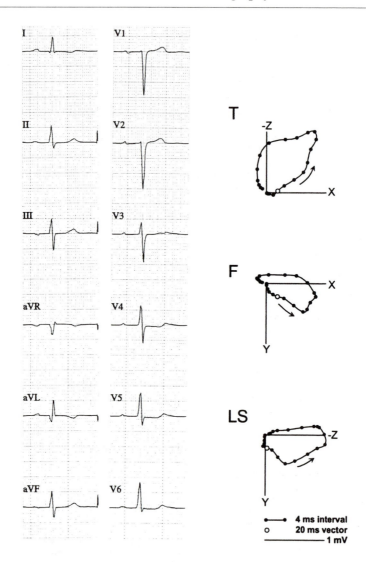

Figure 6.4 *Anterior myocardial infarction proven by diagnostic cardiac catheterization in a 58-year-old male. Note the QRS loop area in the left anterior quadrant is almost zero percent of the total QRS loop area.*

6.2.3 Inferior myocardial infarction

The dead zone or infarct vector concept suggests that in inferior myocardial infarction there is an increase of electrical force superiorly. In turn, this produces a loss of inferiorly directed forces resulting in an initial superiorly directed vectorcardiographic loop in the frontal plane. However, as this is not altogether uncommon in normal individuals, the point of importance is the length of time for which the loop persists in the superior quadrants and the ratio of superiorly to inferiorly directed forces. Common vectorcardiographic criteria for inferior myocardial infarction are presented in Table 6.2.

Table 6.2 Criteria for inferior myocardial infarction.

All of the following in the frontal QRS loop:
an initial superior inscription > 20 ms
a superior amplitude > 0.1 mV
a superior/inferior amplitude ratio > 0.15
an X axis intercept > 0.3 mV

In addition to the superiorly directed forces having a duration > 20 ms, the concept of X intercept needs to be introduced. This is illustrated in Figure 6.5. The X intercept is the point at which a clockwise inscribed frontal plane loop first crosses the X axis. In a sense, it is clear that the longer the QRS loop remains superior to the X axis, then the greater the probability that the X intercept will exceed 0.3 mV. Thus, in some ways there is a correlation between this parameter and a superior duration > 20 ms. Figure 6.6 gives an example of a vectorcardiographic frontal plane loop where all the criteria are met.

Analogous to the situation of low R waves in anterior leads consistent with myocardial infarction, it is possible that there can be very low amplitude R waves in the inferior lead Y in the presence of inferior infarction, i.e. there is a very short inferiorly directed initial activation in the frontal plane. If the initial vector of activation is directed inferiorly and rightwards followed by clockwise inscription, then the criteria of X intercept > 0.3 mV and a superior/inferior amplitude ratio > 0.15 can often be met.

6.2.4 Inferior myocardial infarction versus left anterior fascicular block

Often a common feature of inferior myocardial infarction and left anterior fascicular block is the superior orientation of the frontal plane QRS vector loop. However, left anterior fascicular block is always accompanied by counter-clockwise inscription of the QRS loop whereas inferior myocardial infarction invariably has clockwise inscription of the QRS loop. A comparative example is shown

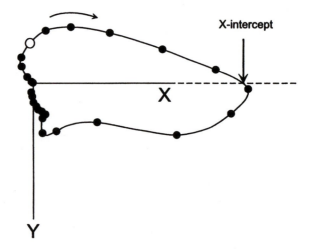

Figure 6.5 *Frontal plane QRS loop showing the X intercept.*

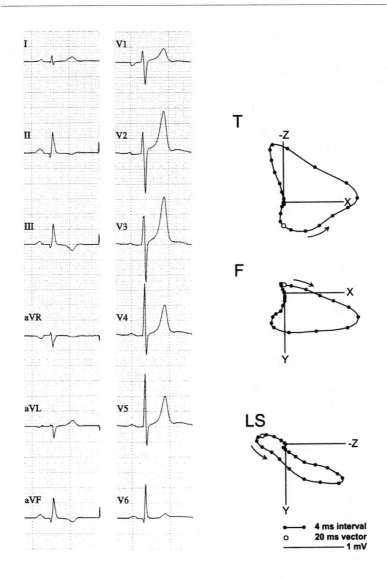

Figure 6.6 *Vectorcardiogram of inferior myocardial infarction meeting the criteria of Table 6.2.*

in Figure 6.7. It is also the case that in left anterior fascicular block, the QRS axis is generally more superiorly directed than in inferior myocardial infarction.

6.2.5 Posterior myocardial infarction

The theory of the dead zone or infarct vector applied to an infarction of the posterior wall of the heart indicates that there will be an increase in anteriorly directed electrical forces. The diagnosis of posterior myocardial infarction is again difficult, purely from an electrocardiographic standpoint. There may, of course, well be other clinical factors that suggest a myocardial infarction which, taken together with the relevant vectorcardiographic changes, could point to infarction of the posterior wall.

The increase in anterior forces is reflected in an increased duration of the anteriorly directed forces in the transverse plane. In addition, the amplitude ratio of the anteriorly/posteriorly directed forces exceeds 1. Finally, the area in the left anterior quadrant of the transverse plane exceeds 50% of the total QRS loop area (Figure 6.8). Common vectorcardiographic criteria for posterior myocardial infarction are presented in Table 6.3.

The other typical feature of posterior myocardial infarction is an increase in T vector amplitude. This may well correspond to a T vector oriented in the direction of $70^{\circ}-80^{\circ}$ in the transverse plane.

Table 6.3 Criteria for posterior myocardial infarction.

The QRS loop in the transverse plane shows:
an initial anteriorly directed loop > 50ms
an anterior/posterior amplitude ratio > 1
a loop area in left anterior quadrant > 50 % of the total loop area

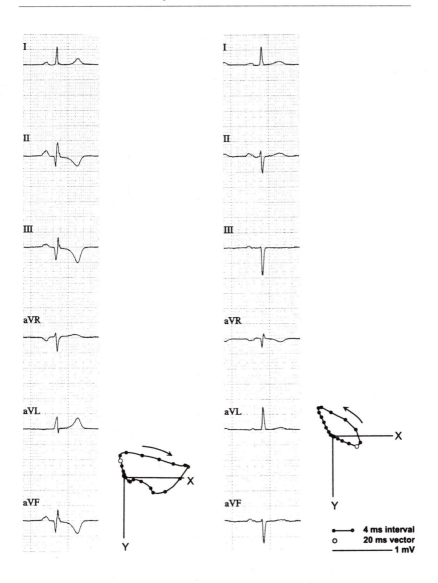

Figure 6.7 *Left panel shows inferior myocardial infarction; right panel shows left anterior fascicular block.*

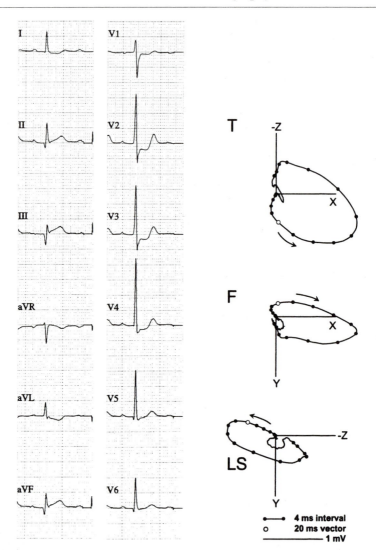

Figure 6.8 *Inferior myocardial infarction with posterior wall involvement. Note that the area of the QRS loop in the left anterior quadrant exceeds 50 % of the total QRS loop area. The X intercept also greatly exceeds 0.3 mV.*

6.2.6 Posterior myocardial infarction versus RVH

The features of RVH have been discussed in Chapter 5. The Type A vectorcardiographic loop is not too dissimilar from that of posterior myocardial infarction and therefore the differentiation between the two is difficult. However, the criteria of anteriorly directed forces exceeding 50 ms is more likely to be met in a case of posterior myocardial infarction than in RVH. Also, the T vector loop is more likely to be anteriorly directed in posterior infarction than in RVH.

One other factor which influences the situation is that inferior or even lateral myocardial infarction which extends towards the posterior wall of the heart, may produce, in addition, an increase in anteriorly directed forces. In that situation, a report of "increased anterior forces probably reflecting inferior/posterior myocardial infarction" is more likely to be correct than one which suggests that there is RVH in addition to inferior infarction, for example.

6.2.7 Anterolateral myocardial infarction

The effect of a lateral wall myocardial infarction is to produce an initial electrical force which is directed in the range $90^{\circ}-270^{\circ}$ in the transverse plane. This is the principal requirement for the diagnosis of anterolateral myocardial infarction, an example of which is shown in Figure 6.9. Isolated anterolateral infarction is uncommon and more often than not, the changes are associated with an anterior rather than a purely anterolateral myocardial infarction.

6.2.8 Bites

The concept of a vectorcardiographic bite was mentioned earlier in the chapter. This is best explained by reference to Figure 6.10 where a comparison is made between a normal transverse plane vectorcardiogram and one exhibiting a bite, i.e. an indentation of the QRS loop which often amounts to a reversal of the direction of inscription of the loop. For example, the normal QRS loop in the transverse plane has a constant counter-clockwise inscription whereas the loop with a bite has an inscription which is initially

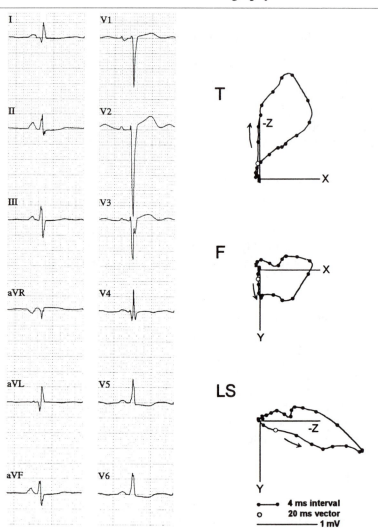

Figure 6.9 Vectorcardiographic example of anterolateral myocardial infarction. Note that in the transverse plane, the initial electrical forces are directed posteriorly to the right and that the inscription of the main body of this loop is clockwise. It should also be noted that there are no Q waves in the precordial leads of the 12-lead ECG.

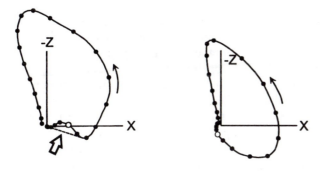

Figure 6.10 *Vectorcardiographic loops in the transverse plane. The left loop shows an early bite whereas the right loop has a normal inscription.*

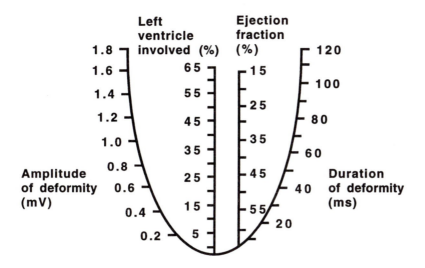

Figure 6.11 *Nomogram for predicting infarct size from deformities in the Frank vectorcardiogram. The amplitude and duration of the deformity are transferred to the left and right side of the nomogram, respectively. A line is then constructed through these two points and the points where it crosses the lines in the centre are used to determine the angiographic percentage of left ventricle involved and the ejection fraction.*

counter-clockwise, then changes to clockwise before returning to counter-clockwise inscription. It is suggested that the amount of deviation of the bite from the normal loop gives an indication of the size of infarcted area. Considerable work was done in this area by Selvester and Sanmarco (1978) with modelling studies and indeed, a nomogram was produced which linked the duration of the bite with the magnitude of the difference between the normal and the abnormal vectorcardiographic loop (Figure 6.11). The nomogram allows calculation of an estimate of the percentage of myocardium which is damaged and in turn, an estimate of the ejection fraction of the left ventricle. Selvester et al. (1968) also provided data on the ocurrence of bites in diabetic patients. Edenbrandt et al. recently (1989) developed a computer assisted method for measuring the size of vectorcardiographic bites.

7 CONDUCTION DEFECTS

7.1 Introduction

It is certainly the case that conduction defects may be thought rather straightforward to diagnose from the 12-lead ECG. On the other hand, there are borderline situations where there can be doubt as to whether a QRS duration is prolonged. Indeed, it has gone almost unrecognised for many years that the normal mean QRS duration for males is almost 8 ms longer than for females in the 18–29 year age group (96.4 versus 87.7 ms) although as age increases the difference tends to decrease (92.7 versus 87.1 ms at 50 years and over) (Macfarlane and Lawrie, 1989a). Notwithstanding this, there are few if any diagnostic criteria which take cognisance of this fact.

One of the advantages of vectorcardiography is that conduction defects can be seen on the vectorcardiographic loop display as a slowing of the inscription of the loop, i.e. the loop markers appear closer together. There are other features sometimes pathognomonic of particular defects, as will be seen later in the Chapter.

7.1.1 Conduction system

The heart muscle consists of three types of tissue – automatic, specialised conducting and contractile tissue. The process of depolarisation is common to all three tissues but only the automatic and specialised conducting tissues have the ability to depolarise spontaneously.

In the human heart (Figure 7.1), the automatic tissue is concentrated mainly at the sinoatrial (SA) node. In the normal sequence of electrical events, an electrical impulse arising in the SA node, travels through the right atrium to the atrioventricular (AV) node and thereafter spreads into the ventricles via the specialised conducting tissue in the bundle of His.

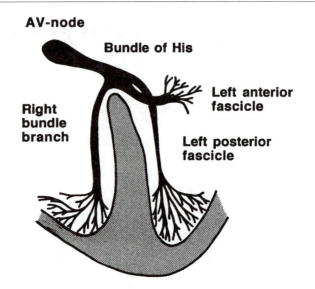

AV-node

Bundle of His

Left anterior fascicle

Right bundle branch

Left posterior fascicle

Figure 7.1 Conduction system of the human heart.

Invasive recording of the signals in the atria and in particular in the area of the AV node has recently led to a much greater understanding of certain types of conduction defects but in particular, this approach has been of most value in the assessment of cardiac arrhythmias. On the other hand, this chapter is concerned more with abnormalities of conduction in the bundle of His and its various branches.

As seen in Figure 7.1, the bundle of His divides at the base of the septum into the right bundle branch and the left bundle branch. The latter has been shown to divide into a variety of different forms, common to all of which are the left anterior and left posterior fascicles. Demoulin and Kulbertus (1972) showed many years ago that there was often a third fascicle which they called 'the centroseptal fascicle'.

Under normal circumstances, ventricular depolarisation occurs first in the left ventricle, particularly on the left side of the septum, and then spreads to the free wall of the left ventricle. At the same time, shortly after left ventricular activation commences, the right ventricular excitation also starts. However, it is important to appreciate that the normal sequence of depolarisation in the ventricles is from the left to the right side of the septum.

For completeness, it should be said that excitation in general terms spreads from the endocardium to the epicardium and from apex to base. In addition, ventricular repolarisation takes place from epicardium to endocardium, giving rise to a normal upright T wave in the majority of precordial leads as well as most frontal plane leads with the exception of aVR. In the 12-lead vectorcardiogram, the T wave is normally upright in leads X, Y and Z.

7.2 Bundle branch block

7.2.1 Left bundle branch block

When the normal conduction to the left ventricle is prevented by a block in the left bundle branch, the excitation wavefront has to find an alternative pathway via normal cardiac muscle. A major consequence of this is naturally an increase in the time taken to depolarise the ventricles and hence, there is an increase in the QRS duration.

Because of the block in the left bundle branch above its division into the various fascicles, septal activation begins on the right side and progresses from right to left. Thus, in the 12-lead vectorcardiogram in left bundle branch block (LBBB), there is frequently no primary R wave in lead Z and almost always, an absence of a Q wave in the anterolateral lead X. Right ventricular depolarisation is virtually complete before the excitation waves later spread unopposed round both anterior and posterior walls of the left ventricle to meet at the lateral wall (van Dam, 1976).

From a vectorcardiographic point of view, the initial QRS forces are therefore directed posteriorly and to the left. Commonly, the maximum QRS vector is also similarly directed posteriorly to the left and inferiorly. The vectorcardiographic appearances of LBBB are as shown in Figure 7.2. These are quite distinctive with generally a long narrow QRS loop in the transverse plane with the T loop being oppositely directed. This corresponds to T wave inversion in lead X. It does also suggest that ventricular repolarisation takes place in a sequence parallel to that of depolarisation in view of the abnormally slow spread of the ventricular activation wave fronts. The characteristic vectorcardiographic features of LBBB are shown in Table 7.1.

Table 7.1 Vectorcardiographic criteria for left bundle branch block.

A maximum QRS vector directed oppositely to the T vector.
An elongated or occasionally figure-of-eight loop in the transverse plane with minimal breadth.
The main body of the loop is usually inscribed in a clockwise direction in the transverse plane.
The timing markers are much closer together than in the normal vectorcardiographic loop.

7.2.2 Incomplete left bundle branch block

The concept of incomplete LBBB is perhaps more difficult to explain. It has been suggested that the progression of excitation via the left bundle branch is slower than normal although there is not a complete block. Initial septal activation will, therefore, be on the right side of the septum. From the vectorcardiographic point of view, the QRS loop is again elongated and narrow as in complete LBBB but the overall QRS duration is of the order of 120-140 ms. The remaining markers may also be a little closer than normal. An illustration is given in Figure 7.3.

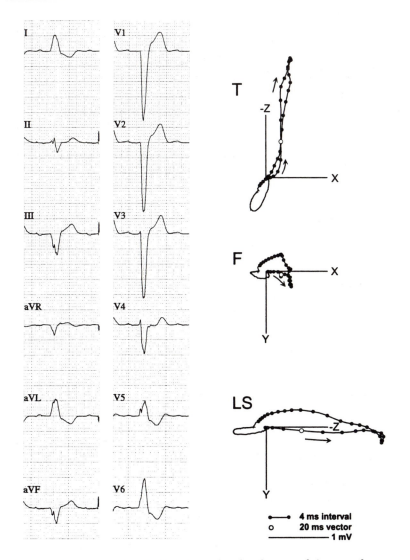

Figure 7.2 An example of LBBB. Note the closely spaced time-markers and the narrowness of the QRS loop particularly in the transverse plane. Also, it should be noted that the maximum QRS and T vectors are oppositely directed.

99

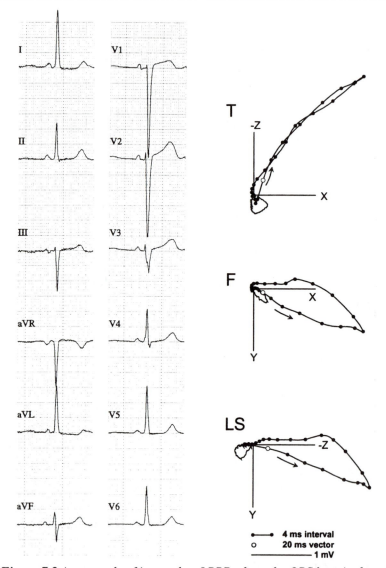

Figure 7.3 *An example of incomplete LBBB where the QRS loop in the transverse plane is extremely narrow. The time-markers are also more closely spaced than normal.*

100

Often this pattern is associated with a slightly increased voltage and T wave abnormalities in the lateral leads, i.e. a T vector loop almost oppositely directed to the QRS loop. This has given rise to the expression 'incomplete LBBB/LVH pattern'. It is possible that patients with hypertensive heart disease, for example, and LVH, exhibit fibrosis which progresses to the extent that the conduction system becomes impaired resulting in the above described abnormalities.

7.2.3 Right bundle branch block

In complete right bundle branch block (RBBB), there is a block in the conduction system in the right bundle branch below its junction with the bundle of His. Thus, left ventricular activation commences normally so that RBBB always manifests itself as an abnormality in the terminal part of the QRS complex. This allows other abnormalities such as myocardial infarction to be reported with reasonable confidence in the presence of RBBB.

Because of the normal left ventricular activation, appearances in RBBB show normal initial depolarisation. After the greater part of the left ventricle has been depolarised, the delayed excitation wave has spread to the free wall of the right ventricle so that there is an electrically unopposed (but delayed) right ventricular depolarisation. This results in the terminal portion of the QRS complex exhibiting electrical forces oriented to the right, anteriorly. In addition, the QRS duration is abnormally prolonged beyond 120 ms. In the scalar presentation of lead Z there is a broad R' wave.

The vectorcardiographic loop is shown in Figure 7.4. It can be seen that the terminal portion of the QRS loop shows a marked slowing of the rate of inscription as evidenced by the closeness of the timing markers. The terminal loop is directed anteriorly, rightwards, with quite characteristic features being demonstrated. The major part of the loop is inscribed in a counter-clockwise direction.

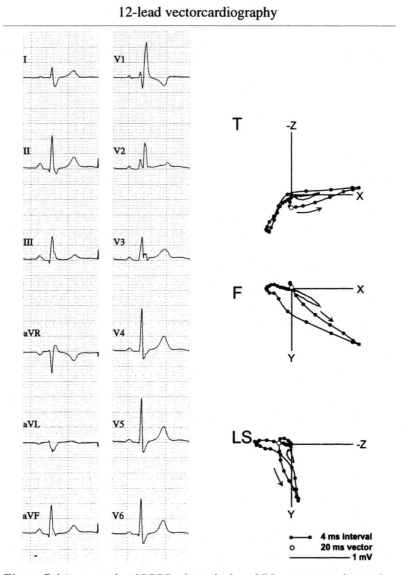

Figure 7.4 *An example of RBBB where the late QRS vectors are directed anteriorly to the right with very closely spaced time-markers in the loops corresponding to the slowed conduction. Note the terminal slowing of inscription of the QRS loop.*

7.2.4 Incomplete right bundle branch block

There can often be dispute as to whether on a scalar presentation there is, indeed, incomplete RBBB evidenced by the secondary r' wave in V_1, V_2 or lead Z. It has been suggested that this late QRS activity is due to hypertrophy of the basal portion of the right ventricle although, as it is often seen in younger individuals, it could indeed on occasions be considered a normal variant.

From the vectorcardiographic point of view, an incomplete RBBB is manifested as some slowing in the terminal inscription of the QRS loop seen best in the transverse plane. This portion of the loop will also be oriented anteriorly, rightwards. In this situation, the presentation of a vectorcardiogram has an advantage over the scalar presentation in that terminal slowing can be seen.

It could be argued, since the normal QRS duration ranges from 60 to 110 ms, that an incomplete bundle branch block occurring in a patient who previously had a QRS duration of the order of 80 ms could well result in a relative prolongation of the QRS duration to 110 ms. Therefore, it should not be essential for conduction defects involving the right bundle branch in particular to be dependent on criteria which provide discrete time thresholds such as 110 ms for incomplete RBBB. On the other hand, it is unlikely in the adult that a QRS duration < 90 ms would be consistent with even an incomplete RBBB. An illustration of the vectorcardiogram in incomplete RBBB is given in Figure 7.5.

7.3 Fascicular block

In 1966, Pryor and Blount suggested that pure left axis deviation might be due to a block in the superior division of the left bundle. They termed this abnormality 'Left Superior Intraventricular Block'. They also suggested that right axis deviation could be caused by a block in the inferior division of the left bundle. It was surmised that the direction of the initial excitation depended on the nature of the lesion which produced the block, e.g. fibrosis or

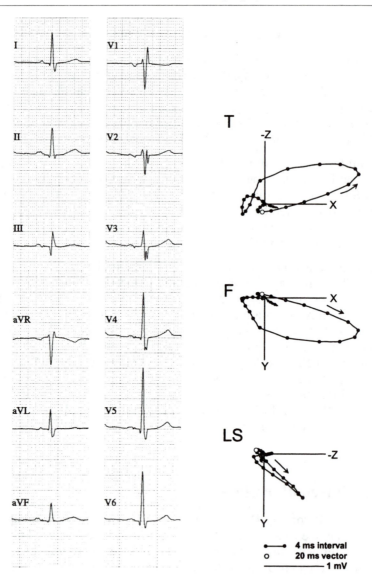

Figure 7.5 *Example of incomplete RBBB.*

necrosis. Subsequently, Rosenbaum (1970) set out criteria for conduction defects arising from different parts of the conducting system. He postulated that localised abnormalities may occur in isolation, intermittently or in association with defects in other branches of the specialised conducting system. He also introduced the term 'hemiblock' to replace 'superior' and 'inferior' intraventricular block but since there are often more than two specialised conducting fascicles in the left ventricle as shown in Figure 7.1, the term is perhaps a misnomer. For this reason, it has been suggested (Pryor, 1972) that the term 'fascicular block' be used. This terminology will be used in the present discussion.

7.3.1 Left anterior fascicular block

In left anterior fascicular block, it is postulated that a block of the conduction of excitation arises in the anterior fascicle of the left bundle branch. In this case, ventricular depolarisation probably takes place via the other intact fascicles. Excitation initially spreads inferiorly from the left posterior fascicle and it is feasible that there may also be some septal activation from another left sided conducting fascicle such as the centroseptal fascicle. The net result is an initial, inferiorly directed and sometimes rightward spread of activation. Thereafter, the leftward upward spread of activation from the region of the left posterior fascicle becomes dominant, causing the ventricular resultant electrical force to be orientated posteriorly and superiorly producing a prominent S wave in lead Y.

The frontal plane vectorcardiographic loop shows left axis deviation in most cases, i.e. the projection of the maximum QRS vector is superior to $0°$ and always has counter-clockwise inscription (Kulbertus et al., 1970). This enables left anterior fascicular block to be differentiated from other forms of conduction abnormality such as due to inferior myocardial infarction. Figure 7.6 gives an example of left anterior fascicular block while Figure 6.7 shows how inferior myocardial infarction can be separated from left anterior fascicular block by the fact that there is clockwise inscription in the frontal plane in the former. Lopes (1974) has proposed that the vectorcar-

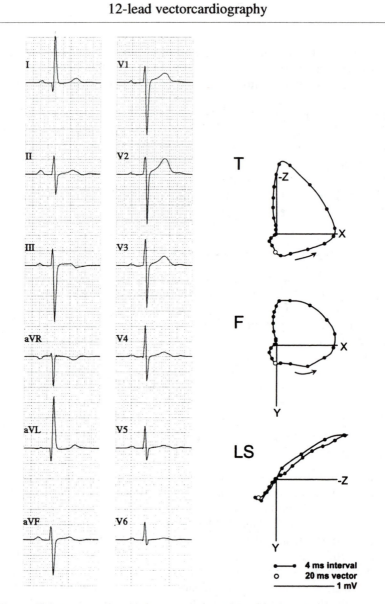

Figure 7.6 *An example of left anterior fascicular block with counter-clockwise inscription of the QRS loop in the frontal plane.*

106

diographic criteria for left anterior fascicular block should include those listed in Table 7.2.

He also suggested that if the major axis of the QRS loop is not directed superiorly, but the late part of the loop lies in the left superior quadrant, possible left anterior fascicular block may be diagnosed.

7.3.2 Left posterior fascicular block

It is postulated that if there is a block in the posterior fascicle of the left bundle branch, ventricular activation will proceed from the anterior wall of the left ventricle, spreading inferiorly. Right ventricular, and possibly septal activation are normal. However, the posterior wall of the left ventricle will be depolarised somewhat later than usual so that the excitation waves spreading anteriorly and inferiorly assume an increased importance in the development of ECG appearances. The QRS axis, therefore, shifts to the right, producing appearances suggestive of RVH. Often these appearances are best seen in an intermittent conduction defect in a rhythm strip, for example (Figure 7.7). In this example, there are atrial extrasystoles which show a change in QRS configuration compared to the dominant complex, namely, an increase in the amplitude of the R wave in the anteroseptal and inferior leads and a deepening of the S wave in the lateral lead. These appearances are in keeping with the concept of left posterior fascicular block which, in this case, is intermittent, presumably being produced by a refractory left posterior fascicle at the time of occurrence of the supraventricular extrasystole.

Table 7.2 Vectorcardiographic criteria for left anterior fascicular block.

Initial QRS vectors directed inferiorly and rightward.
Counter-clockwise inscription in the frontal plane.
QRS axis in the frontal plane superior to -30° .

The differentiation of pure left posterior fascicular block from RVH can be difficult. The former is best diagnosed only if there is a lack of clinical evidence to support RVH. It should be clear from the figure that the diagnosis of pure left posterior fascicular block from a single cardiac cycle is virtually impossible.

7.4 Bifascicular block

Combinations of conduction abnormalities in the right bundle branch and different fascicles of the left bundle branch lead to bifascicular block. An example of bifascicular block is RBBB in association with left anterior fascicular block (Figure 7.8). In this case, there is a marked superior displacement of the vectorcardiographic loop in the frontal plane while the terminal slowing of con-

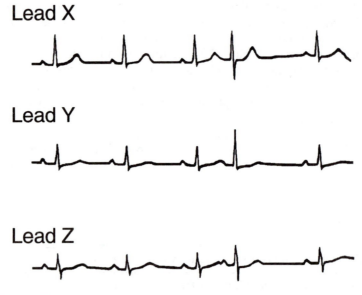

Figure 7.7 *Example of intermittent left posterior fascicular block in the fourth beat.*

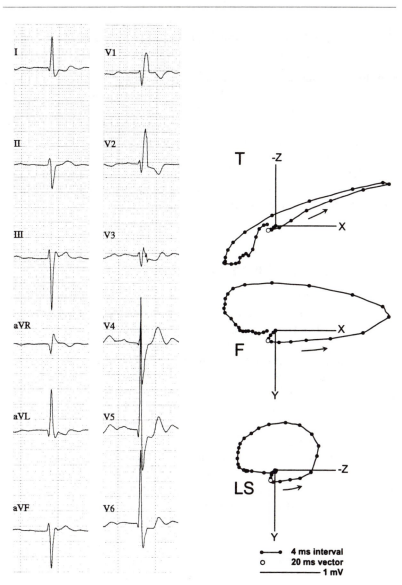

Figure 7.8 Example of RBBB + left anterior fascicular block.

109

duction is again apparent in the transverse plane where the terminal forces are directed anteriorly and to the right.

On the other hand, RBBB with a left posterior fascicular block may be suspected when there is right axis deviation with other typical features of RBBB (Figure 7.9). Again, the typical RBBB feature of terminal slowing of the QRS loop is apparent but the right axis deviation is abnormal. This feature can perhaps be seen more clearly in another rare example (Figure 7.10) where there is electrical alternans. The narrow QRS complex suggests myocardial infarction with possible left posterior fascicular block while the alternate beats indicate RBBB in addition.

7.5 Wolff-Parkinson-White pattern

The classical features of Wolff-Parkinson-White (WPW) (1930) pattern are those of an initial slurring of the QRS complex due to the spread of activation from atria to ventricles via an accessory pathway. Note that these features describe the WPW pattern which, if associated with episodes of paroxysmal tachycardia, gives rise to the WPW syndrome. From the vectorcardiographic point of view, the main distinguishing feature is obviously the slowing of inscription in the initial part of the vectorcardiographic loop. This may facilitate the diagnosis of WPW pattern in borderline cases where the initial slurring in the scalar presentation may be questioned as being technical in origin. There is a variety of accessory pathways such that there is no typical feature of the WPW pattern on the vectorcardiogram other than the initial slowing of inscription. In other words, initial vectors may be orientated in a whole spectrum of different directions depending on the location of the accessory pathway.

In broad terms, using the older classification of Type A and Type B, the initial vector orientation will be anterior in Type A and posterior/to the left in Type B. Figures 7.11 and 7.12 give examples of the vectorcardiographic loops in the WPW pattern.

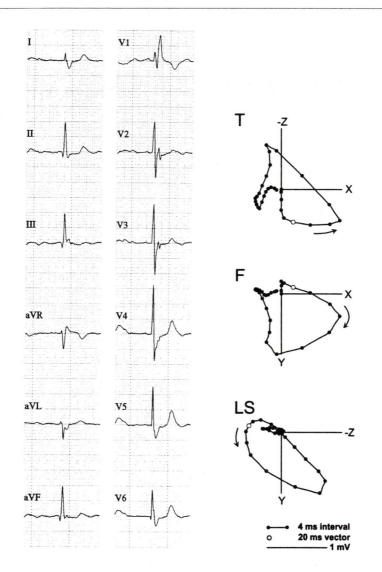

Figure 7.9 *An example of RBBB plus left posterior fascicular block. Note that the QRS vector in the frontal plane exceeds 75° in this 39-year-old male.*

111

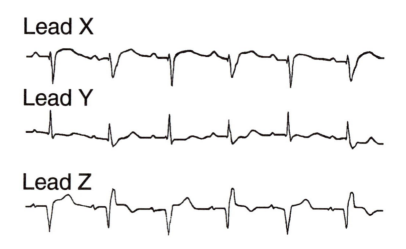

Figure 7.10 *Example of alternans where every second beat shows RBBB plus left posterior fascicular block.*

7.6 Intraventricular conduction defects

There remains a class of conduction defects which do not fit any of the categories mentioned so far. In general terms, the QRS duration is prolonged in excess of 120 ms but the features of RBBB or LBBB are not apparent. On occasions, such defects manifest themselves as an open loop in the transverse plane which permits the diagnosis of intraventricular conduction defect as opposed to LBBB, for example, even when the QRS duration is the order of 140 to 160 ms (Figure 7.13). This is another area where the vectorcardiographic loop can be of considerable diagnostic value.

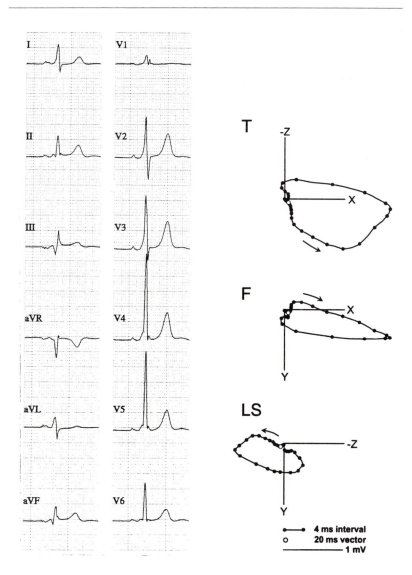

Figure 7.11 *An example of WPW Type A with initial slowing of the inscription of the QRS loop and early QRS vectors directed anteriorly.*

113

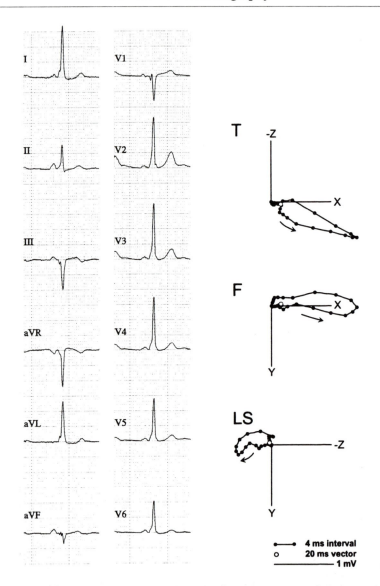

Figure 7.12 *An example of WPW Type B where there is initial slowing of the early QRS vectors which are directed leftwards for the first 20 ms.*

114

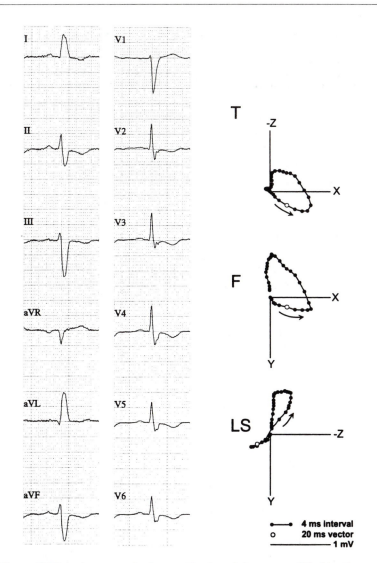

Figure 7.13 *An intraventricular conduction defect exemplified by the closely spaced time-markers in all the QRS loops. The transverse loop is also open as opposed to being narrow in LBBB and does not have the late QRS vectors directed to the right as in RBBB.*

115

7.7 Combined conduction defects and myocardial infarction

The diagnosis of myocardial infarction in the presence of RBBB is relatively straightforward. Because RBBB affects the terminal portion of the QRS complex and classical criteria for myocardial infarction affect the initial portion of the QRS complex, then it is possible for myocardial infarction to be reported in the presence of RBBB. Figure 7.14 shows an example of inferior myocardial infarction and RBBB.

On the other hand, there is still controversy over the diagnosis of myocardial infarction in the presence of LBBB. In 1982, Havelda et al. suggested that inferior myocardial infarction could be diagnosed with 100% specificity in the presence of LBBB given that there were QS complexes in the inferior leads. Others have subsequently suggested that anterior infarction can be diagnosed in the presence of LBBB when, for example, there is a reversed R wave progression from V_3 to V_5 or there are Q waves in the lateral leads. On the other hand, left anterior fascicular block may mask or mimic inferior infarction (Milliken 1983).

7.8 ECG versus 12-lead vectorcardiogram in conduction defects

This chapter has shown how there are certain situations where the vectorcardiographic display can exhibit the presence of conduction defects which may be less obvious on the scalar ECG. In particular, the slowing of timing marks on the vectorcardiogram is invariably an illustration of a conduction defect, whether it be at the beginning of the QRS complex as in the WPW pattern or at the end as in RBBB. If the slowing is throughout the QRS, then most likely the diagnosis is LBBB. It has also been shown how left anterior fascicular block and inferior infarction can be separated by the direction of inscription of the frontal plane vectorcardiographic loop. All of

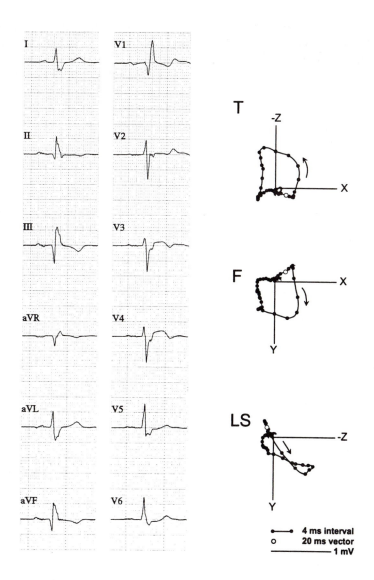

Figure 7.14 *Example of RBBB and inferior myocardial infarction.*

these points lend further weight to the conclusion that the vector-cardiogram has an important role to play in the diagnosis of ventricular conduction defects.

REFERENCES

American College of Cardiology, 10th Bethesda conference report on optimal electrocardiology. Am J Cardiol 1978;41:111–191.

American Heart Association and the Cardiac Society of Great Britain and Ireland. Committee for the standardisation of precordial leads. Supplementary report. Am Heart J 1938;15:107–108, 235–239.

American Heart Association. Committee for the standardization of precordial leads. Second supplementary report. JAMA 1943;121:1349–1351.

American Heart Association. Committee on Electrocardiography (Pipberger HV, Arzbaecher RC, Berson AS, et al.). Recommendations for standardization of leads and of specifications for instruments in electrocardiography and vectorcardiography. Circulation 1975;52(Suppl):11–31.

Bjerle P, Arvedson O. Comparison of Frank vectorcardiogram with two different vectorcardiograms derived from conventional ECG-leads. Proc Eng Found Conf 1986;11:13–26.

Bonner RE, Crevasse L, Ferrer MI, Greenfield JC. A new computer program for analysis of scalar electrocardiograms. Comput Biomed Res 1972;5:629–653.

Brohet CR. Special value of the vectorcardiogram in pediatric cardiology. J Electrocardiol 1990;23(Suppl):58–62.

Caceres CA, Steinberg CA, Abraham S, et al. Computer extraction of electrocardiographic parameters. Circulation 1962;25:356–362.

Chen CY, Chiang BN, Macfarlane PW. Normal limits of the electrocardiogram in a Chinese population. J Electrocardiol 1989;22:1–15.

Chou T, Helm RA. The pseudo P pulmonale. Circulation, 1965;32:96–105.

Demoulin JC, Kulbertus HE. Histopathological examination of the concept of left hemiblock. Br Heart J 1972;34:807–814.

Dower GE, Machado HB, Osborne JA. On deriving the electrocardiogram from vectorcardiographic leads. Clin Cardiol 1980;3:87–95.

Downs TD, Liebman J, Agusti R, Romberg HC. The statistical treatment of angular data in vectorcardiography. In: Hoffman I, Traymore RC, eds. Proc. Long Island Jewish Hospital Symposium on Vectorcardiography, 1965. Amsterdam: North Holland, 1966:272–278.

Draper HW, Peffer CJ, Stallmann FW, Littmann D, Pipberger HV. The corrected orthogonal electrocardiogram and vectorcardiogram in 510 normal men (Frank lead system). Circulation 1964;30:853–864.

Edenbrandt L, Pahlm O. Vectorcardiogram synthesized from a 12-lead ECG: superiority of the inverse Dower matrix. J Electrocardiol 1988;21:361–367.

Edenbrandt L, Ek A, Lundh B, Pahlm O. Vectorcardiographic bites. A method for detection and quantification applied on a normal material. J Electrocardiol 1989;22:325–331.

Edenbrandt L, Houston A, Macfarlane PW. Vectorcardiograms synthesized from 12-lead ECGs: a new method applied in 1,792 healthy children. Pediatr Cardiol 1994;15:21–26.

Einthoven W. Weiters über das Elektrokardiogramm. Pflügers Arch. 1908;122:517–584.

Einthoven W. The different forms of the human electrocardiogram and their signification. Lancet 1912;1:853–861.

References

Einthoven W, Fahr G, de Waart A. Über die Richtung und die manifeste Grosse der Potentialschwankungen im menschlichen Herzen und über den Einfluss der Herzlage auf die Form des Elektrokardiogramms. Pflügers Arch 1913;150:175–315. (Translation: Hoff HE, Sekelj P. Am Heart J 1957;40:163–194)

Frank E. A direct experimental study of three systems of spatial vectorcardiography. Circulation 1954a;10:101–113.

Frank E. The image surface of a homogeneous torso. Am Heart J 1954b;47:757–768.

Frank E. An accurate, clinically practical system for spatial vectorcardiography. Circulation, 1956;13:737–749.

Goldberger E. A simple, indifferent, electrocardiographic electrode of zero potential and a technique of obtaining augmented unipolar, extremity leads. Am Heart J 1942;23:483–492.

Gottdiener JS, Gay JA, Maron BJ, Fletcher RD. Increased right ventricular wall thickness in left ventricular pressure overload: Echocardiographic determination of hypertrophic response of the 'non-stressed' ventricle. J Am Coll Cardiol 1985;6:550–555.

Grishman A, Scherlis L. Spatial vectorcardiography. Philadelphia: Saunders, 1952.

Havelda CLJ, Sohi GS, Flowers NC, Horan LG. The pathologic correlates of the electrocardiogram: Complete left bundle branch block. Circulation 1982;65:445–451.

Huwez FU. Electrocardiography of the left ventricle in coronary artery disease and hypertrophy. Ph.D. Thesis: University of Glasgow, 1990.

Huwez FU, Pringle SD, Macfarlane PW. A new classification of left ventricular geometry in patients with cardiac disease based on M-Mode echocardiography. Am J Cardiol 1992;70:681–688.

Kannel WB. Prevalence and natural history of electrocardiographic left ventricular hypertrophy. Am J Med 1983;75(Suppl 3A):4–11.

Kors JA, van Herpen G, Sittig AC, van Bemmel JH. Reconstruction of the Frank vectorcardiogram from standard electrocardiographic leads: Diagnostic comparison of different methods. Eur Heart J 1990;11:1083–92.

Kulbertus HE, Collignon P, Humblet L.Vectorcardiographic study of the QRS loop in patients with left anterior focal block. Am Heart J 1970;79:293–304.

Lewis T. The mechanism and graphic registration of the heart beat. 3rd edn. London: Shaw, 1925.

Lopes MG. Seminar in vectorcardiography. Stanford, California: Stanford University Press, 1974.

Lundh B. On the normal scalar ECG. A new classification system considering age, sex and heart position. Acta Med Scand 1984;suppl. 691.

Macfarlane PW, Lorimer AR, Lawrie TDV. 3- and 12-lead electro-cardiogram interpretation by computer. A comparison of 1093 patients. Br Heart J 1971;33:266–274.

Macfarlane PW. British Regional Heart Study: The electrocardio-gram and risk of myocardial infarction on follow-up. J Electrocar-diol 1987;20(Suppl):53–56.

Macfarlane PW, Lawrie TDV. The normal electrocardiogram and vectorcardiogram. In: Macfarlane PW, Lawrie TDV, eds. Compre-hensive electrocardiology. Vol 1. Oxford: Pergamon Press, 1989a:407–58.

Macfarlane PW, Coleman EN, Pomphrey EO, McLaughlin S, Hou-ston A. Normal limits of the high-fidelity pediatric ECG. J Electro-cardiol 1989b;22(Suppl):162–168.

Macfarlane PW, Devine B, Latif S, McLaughlin S, Shoat DB, Watts MP. Methodology of ECG interpretation in the Glasgow Program. Meth Inform Med 1990a;29:354–361.

Macfarlane PW, Coleman EN, Devine B, et al. A new 12-lead pediatric ECG interpretation program. J Electrocardiol 1990b;23(Suppl):76–81.

Mann H. A method for analyzing the electrocardiogram. Arch Int Med 1920;25:283–294.

Marquette Electronics Inc., Milwaukee, Wisconsin, USA. Computerising the Heart Station. Physicians' Guide.

Milliken JA. Isolated and complicated left anterior fascicular block: a review of suggested electrocardiographic criteria. J Electrocardiol 1983;16:199–211.

Namin EP, Arcilla RA, D'Cruz IA, Gasul BM. Evaluation of the Frank vectorcardiogram in normal infants. Am J Cardiol 1964;13:757.

Nemati M, Doyle JT, McCaughan D, Dunn RA, Pipberger HV. The orthogonal electrocardiogram in normal women. Implications of sex differences in diagnostic electrocardiography. Am Heart J 1978;95:12–21.

Pipberger HV, Arms RJ, Stallmann FW. Automatic screening of normal and abnormal electrocardiograms by means of a digital electronic computer. Circ Res 1961a;9:1138–1143.

Pipberger HV, Bialek SM, Perloff JK, Schnaper HW. Correlation of clinical information in the standard 12-lead ECG and in a corrected orthogonal 3-lead ECG. Am Heart J 1961b;61:34.

Pryor R. Fascicular blocks and the bilateral bundle branch block syndrome. Am Heart J 1972;83:441.

Pryor R, Blount SG. The clinical significance of true left axis deviation. Am Heart J 1966;72:391–413.

Rosenbaum BM. The hemiblocks: diagnostic criteria and clinical significance. Mod Concepts Cardiovasc Dis 1970;39:141–146.

Rubel P, Benhadid I, Fayn J. Quantitative assessment of eight different methods for synthesizing Frank VCGs from simultaneously recorded standard ECG leads. J Electrocardiol 1991;24(suppl):197–202.

Selvester RH, Rubin HB, Hamlin JA, Pote WW. New quantitative vectorcardiographic criteria for the detection of unsuspected myocardial infarction in diabetics. Am Heart J 1968;75:335–348.

Selvester RH, Sanmarco ME. Infarct size in hi-gain hi-fidelity VCG's and serial ventriculograms in patients with proven coronary artery disease. In: Antoloczy Z, ed. Modern electrocardiology. Amersterdam: Excerpta Medica, 1978:523–528.

Waller AD. A demonstration on man of electromotive changes accompanying the heart's beat. J Physiol 1887;8:229–234.

van Dam R Th. Ventricular activation in human and canine bundle branch block. In: Wellens HJJ, Lie KI, Janse MJ, eds. The conduction system of the heart. Leiden: Stenfert Kroese, 1976:377–392.

Watts MP, Shoat DB. Trends in electrocardiograph design. J Ins Electron Radio Eng 1987;57:140–150.

Willems JL, Poblete PF, Pipberger HV. Day-to-day variation of the normal orthogonal electrocardiogram and vectorcardiogram. Circulation 1972;45:1057–1064.

Wilson FN, Macleod AG, Barker PS. Electrocardiographic leads which record potential variations produced by the heart beat at a single point. Proc Soc Exp Biol Med 1932;29:1011–1012.

Wolff L, Parkinson J, White PD. Bundle-branch block with short P-R interval in healthy young people prone to paroxysmal tachycardia. Am Heart J 1930;5:685–704.

Yang TF, Chen CY, Chiang BN, Macfarlane PW. Normal limits of derived vectorcardiogram in Chinese. J Electrocardiol 1993;26:97–106.

Yang TF, Macfarlane PW. Comparison of the derived vectorcardiogram in apparently healthy Caucasians and Chinese. Chest 1994 (In press)

APPENDIX 1

Normal limits of adult 12-lead vectorcardiogram

The tables of amplitudes and durations in this Appendix have been obtained from the X, Y, Z leads derived from the 12-lead ECG according to the methods described in 3.3.4 and using the coefficients presented in Table 3.2. Data have been derived from 1,555 adult ECGs whose age distribution is shown in the lower part of Table 4.1. The 215 males over 50 have been subdivided, with 38 men being aged 60 and over, while similarly the 139 females include 19 aged 60 and over.

Data are expressed as mean $\pm$ standard deviation below which is given the 96 percentile ranges, i.e. 2% of values are excluded at either end of the distribution except in the case of the groups aged 60 and over where the 100% range is presented. Angular data are presented with respect to the reference frames illustrated in Figure 2.9.

Scalar measurements from the leads X, Y and Z

Table A-D   P wave amplitude and duration

Table E-H   Q wave amplitude and duration

Table I-L   R wave amplitude and duration

Table M-P   S wave amplitude and duration

Table Q-R   T wave amplitude

Planar and spatial measurements

Table S-T   Direction of inscription of the QRS vector loop

Table U   Magnitude of maximal spatial QRS vector

Table V-W   Magnitude of maximal planar QRS vector

Table X-Y   Maximal planar QRS vector angle

Table Z-AA Maximal T vector angle

127

Table A: P wave amplitudes (mV) in males.

Age (years)	X	Y	Z
18–29	0.07 ± 0.02 0.03 → 0.12	0.11 ± 0.05 0.02 → 0.25	0.05 ± 0.02 0.02 → 0.10
30–39	0.07 ± 0.02 0.03 → 0.12	0.11 ± 0.04 0.01 → 0.22	0.04 ± 0.02 0.01 → 0.11
40–49	0.07 ± 0.02 0.03 → 0.14	0.11 ± 0.04 0.03 → 0.22	0.04 ± 0.02 0.00 → 0.09
50–59	0.07 ± 0.02 0.04 → 0.13	0.11 ± 0.04 0.04 → 0.20	0.04 ± 0.02 0.01 → 0.08
60–	0.07 ± 0.03 0.03 → 0.11	0.11 ± 0.04 0.04 → 0.18	0.04 ± 0.03 0.00 → 0.08

Table B: P wave amplitudes (mV) in females.

Age (years)	X	Y	Z
18–29	0.07 ± 0.02 0.03 → 0.13	0.11 ± 0.05 0.02 → 0.26	0.04 ± 0.02 0.01 → 0.08
30–39	0.08 ± 0.02 0.04 → 0.13	0.12 ± 0.05 0.03 → 0.24	0.04 ± 0.02 0.01 → 0.09
40–49	0.08 ± 0.02 0.04 → 0.12	0.11 ± 0.04 0.03 → 0.24	0.04 ± 0.02 0.01 → 0.08
50–59	0.08 ± 0.02 0.04 → 0.13	0.11 ± 0.04 0.03 → 0.22	0.04 ± 0.02 0.00 → 0.07
60–	0.08 ± 0.03 0.03 → 0.14	0.12 ± 0.06 0.03 → 0.23	0.04 ± 0.01 0.01 → 0.06

Table C: P wave durations (ms) in males.

Age (years)	X	Y	Z
18–29	93 ± 14 66 → 122	98 ± 14 66 → 122	98 ± 14 66 → 122
30–39	103 ± 11 78 → 124	103 ± 11 78 → 124	103 ± 11 78 → 124
40–49	107 ± 11 86 → 128	107 ± 11 86 → 128	107 ± 11 86 → 128
50–59	108 ± 11 80 → 128	108 ± 11 80 → 128	108 ± 11 80 → 128
60–	110 ± 12 90 → 130	110 ± 12 90 → 130	110 ± 12 90 → 130

Table D: P wave durations (ms) in females.

Age (years)	X	Y	Z
18–29	97 ± 11 72 → 116	97 ± 11 72 → 116	97 ± 11 72 → 116
30–39	100 ± 10 78 → 116	100 ± 10 78 → 116	100 ± 10 78 → 116
40–49	104 ± 10 82 → 124	104 ± 10 82 → 124	104 ± 10 82 → 124
50–59	104 ± 13 64 → 128	104 ± 13 64 → 128	104 ± 13 64 → 128
60–	104 ± 12 88 → 130	104 ± 12 88 → 130	104 ± 12 88 → 130

Table E: Q wave amplitudes (mV) in males.

Age (years)	X	Y
18–29	-0.11 ± 0.09 -0.37 → -0.02	-0.10 ± 0.06 -0.29 → -0.02
30–39	-0.09 ± 0.08 -0.33 → -0.02	-0.10 ± 0.06 -0.30 → -0.02
40–49	-0.08 ± 0.05 -0.21 → -0.02	-0.07 ± 0.04 -0.17 → -0.02
50–59	-0.09 ± 0.06 -0.26 → -0.02	-0.07 ± 0.05 -0.21 → -0.02
60–	-0.07 ± 0.04 -0.14 → -0.02	-0.08 ± 0.05 -0.21 → -0.02

Table F: Q wave amplitudes (mV) in females.

Age (years)	X	Y
18–29	-0.08 ± 0.06 -0.25 → -0.02	-0.10 ± 0.06 -0.29 → -0.02
30–39	-0.09 ± 0.06 -0.26 → -0.02	-0.08 ± 0.05 -0.20 → -0.02
40–49	-0.07 ± 0.05 -0.22 → -0.02	-0.06 ± 0.03 -0.13 → -0.02
50–59	-0.06 ± 0.04 -0.17 → -0.02	-0.06 ± 0.03 -0.16 → -0.02
60–	-0.07 ± 0.04 -0.14 → -0.02	-0.05 ± 0.03 -0.10 → -0.03

Table G: Q wave durations (ms) in males.

Age (years)	X	Y
18–29	17 ± 5 $8 \rightarrow 28$	19 ± 7 $8 \rightarrow 27$
30–39	16 ± 6 $8 \rightarrow 27$	19 ± 5 $7 \rightarrow 31$
40–49	16 ± 4 $7 \rightarrow 23$	17 ± 5 $6 \rightarrow 25$
50–59	16 ± 4 $10 \rightarrow 24$	18 ± 5 $6 \rightarrow 27$
60–	15 ± 3 $10 \rightarrow 23$	19 ± 5 $5 \rightarrow 29$

Table H: Q wave durations (ms) in females.

Age (years)	X	Y
18–29	15 ± 4 $7 \rightarrow 25$	17 ± 5 $7 \rightarrow 26$
30–39	16 ± 4 $7 \rightarrow 24$	16 ± 4 $6 \rightarrow 24$
40–49	15 ± 3 $9 \rightarrow 21$	14 ± 4 $8 \rightarrow 24$
50–59	14 ± 4 $7 \rightarrow 22$	16 ± 4 $8 \rightarrow 24$
60–	15 ± 4 $9 \rightarrow 24$	13 ± 6 $5 \rightarrow 21$

Table I: R wave amplitudes (mV) in males.

Age (years)	X	Y	Z
18–29	1.66 ± 0.46 0.80 → 2.86	1.16 ± 0.46 0.31 → 2.23	0.52 ± 0.23 0.13 → 1.02
30–39	1.53 ± 0.43 0.69 → 2.44	0.91 ± 0.46 0.14 → 2.13	0.42 ± 0.24 0.09 → 1.07
40–49	1.40 ± 0.43 0.66 → 2.41	0.69 ± 0.39 0.04 → 1.51	0.37 ± 0.19 0.04 → 0.87
50–59	1.38 ± 0.38 0.72 → 2.01	0.58 ± 0.34 0.11 → 1.46	0.36 ± 0.17 0.10 → 0.76
60–	1.20 ± 0.36 0.75 → 1.93	0.65 ± 0.39 0.08 → 1.50	0.30 ± 0.19 0.05 → 0.67

Table J: R wave amplitudes (mV) in females.

Age (years)	X	Y	Z
18–29	1.23 ± 0.34 0.56 → 1.96	0.91 ± 0.34 0.32 → 1.75	0.33 ± 0.15 0.07 → 0.70
30–39	1.23 ± 0.37 0.58 → 1.97	0.87 ± 0.32 0.29 → 1.48	0.32 ± 0.15 0.10 → 0.67
40–49	1.11 ± 0.32 0.62 → 1.75	0.66 ± 0.26 0.24 → 1.16	0.25 ± 0.12 0.04 → 0.49
50–59	1.11 ± 0.29 0.60 → 1.76	0.61 ± 0.31 0.14 → 1.31	0.26 ± 0.14 0.04 → 0.73
60–	1.28 ± 0.46 0.54 → 2.23	0.55 ± 0.21 0.25 → 1.16	0.32 ± 0.14 0.04 → 0.56

Table K: R wave durations (ms) in males.

Age (years)	X	Y	Z
18–29	45 ± 15 27 → 79	55 ± 17 28 → 86	32 ± 9 20 → 45
30–39	46 ± 14 28 → 84	57 ± 16 26 → 86	31 ± 9 17 → 44
40–49	47 ± 14 31 → 82	55 ± 18 15 → 90	32 ± 8 15 → 48
50–59	46 ± 14 30 → 79	55 ± 17 22 → 90	33 ± 8 21 → 52
60–	43 ± 11 29 → 62	54 ± 15 34 → 86	29 ± 8 14 → 40

Table L: R wave durations (ms) in females.

Age (years)	X	Y	Z
18–29	44 ± 12 27 → 76	47 ± 13 24 → 78	28 ± 6 15 → 41
30–39	44 ± 12 31 → 67	48 ± 12 31 → 72	28 ± 5 17 → 38
40–49	45 ± 11 31 → 71	52 ± 14 28 → 86	27 ± 7 10 → 41
50–59	44 ± 11 26 → 86	52 ± 15 20 → 77	27 ± 7 11 → 43
60–	44 ± 11 28 → 64	51 ± 13 33 → 72	32 ± 5 24 → 46

Table M: S wave amplitudes (mV) in males.

Age (years)	X	Y	Z
18–29	-0.27 ± 0.18 $-0.68 \rightarrow -0.05$	-0.16 ± 0.09 $-0.41 \rightarrow -0.03$	-1.38 ± 0.47 $-2.50 \rightarrow -0.59$
30–39	-0.26 ± 0.20 $-0.71 \rightarrow -0.05$	-0.18 ± 0.16 $-0.44 \rightarrow -0.04$	-1.05 ± 0.37 $-1.70 \rightarrow -0.49$
40–49	-0.29 ± 0.18 $-0.73 \rightarrow -0.06$	-0.17 ± 0.13 $-0.44 \rightarrow -0.03$	-0.99 ± 0.35 $-1.52 \rightarrow -0.41$
50–59	-0.25 ± 0.17 $-0.68 \rightarrow -0.04$	-0.17 ± 0.16 $-0.60 \rightarrow -0.05$	-0.87 ± 0.32 $-1.39 \rightarrow -0.31$
60–	-0.35 ± 0.18 $-0.54 \rightarrow -0.17$	-0.18 ± 0.14 $-0.28 \rightarrow -0.06$	-0.81 ± 0.31 $-1.04 \rightarrow -0.48$

Table N: S wave amplitudes (mV) in females.

Age (years)	X	Y	Z
18–29	-0.17 ± 0.10 $-0.52 \rightarrow -0.05$	-0.15 ± 0.09 $-0.42 \rightarrow -0.04$	-0.92 ± 0.34 $-1.65 \rightarrow -0.35$
30–39	-0.20 ± 0.11 $-0.39 \rightarrow -0.06$	-0.14 ± 0.12 $-0.36 \rightarrow -0.05$	-0.92 ± 0.33 $-1.65 \rightarrow -0.35$
40–49	-0.18 ± 0.14 $-0.34 \rightarrow -0.04$	-0.14 ± 0.11 $-0.25 \rightarrow -0.04$	-0.99 ± 0.39 $-1.54 \rightarrow -0.46$
50–59	-0.20 ± 0.14 $-0.42 \rightarrow -0.06$	-0.16 ± 0.09 $-0.29 \rightarrow -0.06$	-0.74 ± 0.30 $-1.32 \rightarrow -0.34$
60–	-0.16 ± 0.10 $-0.19 \rightarrow -0.11$	-0.18 ± 0.10 $-0.17 \rightarrow -0.12$	-0.66 ± 0.25 $-0.79 \rightarrow -0.50$

Table O: S wave durations (ms) in males.

Age (years)	X	Y	Z
18–29	26 ± 12 6 → 48	26 ± 10 7 → 48	53 ± 8 35 → 71
30–39	28 ± 13 7 → 57	29 ± 14 8 → 60	54 ± 10 31 → 71
40–49	31 ± 12 10 → 55	32 ± 15 7 → 68	52 ± 11 25 → 70
50–59	32 ± 12 11 → 53	30 ± 15 8 → 67	50 ± 11 27 → 73
60–	33 ± 12 12 → 56	28 ± 11 11 → 50	53 ± 9 31 → 67

Table P: S wave durations (ms) in females.

Age (years)	X	Y	Z
18–29	24 ± 9 7 → 41	25 ± 9 10 → 45	51 ± 9 30 → 67
30–39	28 ± 9 8 → 43	23 ± 10 8 → 43	52 ± 8 35 → 64
40–49	26 ± 10 12 → 41	26 ± 10 12 → 50	52 ± 8 27 → 75
50–59	27 ± 10 12 → 47	27 ± 11 11 → 58	51 ± 9 30 → 64
60–	29 ± 11 13 → 53	33 ± 15 12 → 50	47 ± 10 20 → 59

Table Q: T wave amplitudes (mV) in males.

Age (years)	X	Y	Z
18–29	0.46 ± 0.19 0.10 → 0.95	0.25 ± 0.11 0.02→0.55	0.47 ± 0.18 0.14 → 0.86
30–39	0.42 ± 0.16 0.12 → 0.80	0.21 ± 0.10 0.03 → 0.48	0.42 ± 0.16 0.08 → 0.80
40–49	0.38 ± 0.17 0.08 → 0.82	0.19 ± 0.10 0.03 → 0.43	0.39 ± 0.15 0.12 → 0.72
50–59	0.35 ± 0.16 0.09 → 0.72	0.17 ± 0.08 0.04 → 0.38	0.38 ± 0.16 0.07 → 0.74
60–	0.36 ± 0.18 0.06 → 0.66	0.21 ± 0.12 0.08 → 0.38	0.33 ± 0.17 0.12 → 0.73

Table R: T wave amplitudes (mV) in females.

Age (years)	X	Y	Z
18–29	0.34 ± 0.12 0.14 → 0.60	0.20 ± 0.08 0.04→0.46	0.23 ± 0.11 0.04 → 0.56
30–39	0.33 ± 0.13 0.12 → 0.64	0.18 ± 0.08 0.05 → 0.37	0.22 ± 0.11 0.02 → 0.43
40–49	0.28 ± 0.11 0.05 → 0.51	0.16 ± 0.07 0.05 → 0.33	0.20 ± 0.09 0.06 → 0.43
50–59	0.27 ± 0.11 0.07 → 0.56	0.17 ± 0.07 0.03 → 0.32	0.20 ± 0.09 0.03 → 0.36
60–	0.26 ± 0.14 0.03 → 0.62	0.17 ± 0.08 0.10 → 0.30	0.21 ± 0.08 0.04 → 0.37

Table S: Direction of inscription of the QRS vector loop in males.

	Frontal	Left Sagittal	Transverse
Counterclockwise	22.9	88.0	98.1
Figure of 8	19.1	8.4	0.9
Clockwise	58.0	3.6	1.0

Table T: Direction of inscription of the QRS vector loop in females

	Frontal	Left Sagittal	Transverse
Counterclockwise	21.8	94.5	97.9
Figure of 8	25.3	3.9	1.2
Clockwise	52.9	1.6	0.9

Table U: Magnitude of maximal spatial QRS vector (mV).

Age (years)	Males	Females
18–29	2.39 ± 0.62 $1.07 \rightarrow 3.97$	1.76 ± 0.47 $0.75 \rightarrow 3.06$
30–39	2.07 ± 0.58 $1.00 \rightarrow 3.61$	1.74 ± 0.46 $0.92 \rightarrow 2.77$
40–49	1.79 ± 0.49 $0.85 \rightarrow 2.94$	1.46 ± 0.41 $0.79 \rightarrow 2.26$
50–59	1.65 ± 0.45 $0.86 \rightarrow 2.91$	1.46 ± 0.37 $0.78 \rightarrow 2.22$
60–	1.57 ± 0.42 $0.99 \rightarrow 2.20$	1.37 ± 0.51 $1.00 \rightarrow 1.90$

Table V: Magnitude of the maximal QRS vector in frontal, sagittal and transverse planes (mV) in males.

Age (years)	Frontal	Sagittal	Transverse
18–29	2.04 ± 0.52 0.99 → 3.26	1.75 ± 0.60 0.70→3.41	2.09 ± 0.52 1.02 → 3.39
30–39	1.80 ± 0.49 0.82 → 3.03	1.48 ± 0.58 0.52 →3.11	1.85 ± 0.48 0.92 → 2.95
40–49	1.59 ± 0.46 0.69 → 2.82	1.23 ± 0.45 0.45 → 2.26	1.64 ± 0.43 0.83 → 2.78
50–59	1.50 ± 0.42 0.77 → 2.70	1.07 ± 0.40 0.44 → 2.05	1.54 ± 0.39 0.84 → 2.76
60–	1.40 ± 0.37 0.92 → 2.03	1.12 ± 0.41 0.64 → 1.91	1.42 ± 0.36 0.89 → 2.08

Table W: Magnitude of the maximal QRS vector in frontal, sagittal and transverse planes (mV) in females.

Age (years)	Frontal	Sagittal	Transverse
18–29	1.54 ± 0.40 0.67 → 2.56	1.28 ± 0.44 0.49→2.48	1.51 ± 0.39 0.67 → 2.58
30–39	1.51 ± 0.42 0.62 → 2.42	1.25 ± 0.43 0.60 →2.25	1.50 ± 0.40 0.88 → 2.51
40–49	1.29 ± 0.37 0.74 → 2.07	1.02 ± 0.35 0.40 → 1.78	1.31 ± 0.36 0.84 → 2.76
50–59	1.29 ± 0.33 0.68 →1.96	1.02 ± 0.36 0.42 → 1.86	1.31 ± 0.31 0.69 → 2.01
60–	1.27 ± 0.52 0.99 → 1.88	0.82 ± 0.30 0.60 → 1.18	1.27 ± 0.48 0.93 → 1.77

Table X: 96-percentile ranges of maximal QRS vector angle (degrees) in males.

Age (years)	Frontal	Sagittal	Transverse
18–29	34 ± 14 $12 \rightarrow 62$	40 ± 24 $0 \rightarrow 96$	-37 ± 26 $-105 \rightarrow 14$
30–39	28 ± 14 $3 \rightarrow 54$	38 ± 36 $-12 \rightarrow 144$	-32 ± 28 $-99 \rightarrow 19$
40–49	23 ± 19 $-2 \rightarrow 53$	33 ± 34 $-13 \rightarrow 140$	-28 ± 31 $-103 \rightarrow 27$
50–59	20 ± 13 $-5 \rightarrow 43$	31 ± 41 $-23 \rightarrow 150$	-25 ± 36 $-117 \rightarrow 25$
60–	22 ± 35 $0 \rightarrow 58$	32 ± 33 $0 \rightarrow 84$	-32 ± 35 $-103 \rightarrow 25$

Table Y: 96-percentile ranges of maximal QRS vector angle (degrees) in females.

Age (years)	Frontal	Sagittal	Transverse
18–29	34 ± 15 $13 \rightarrow 59$	44 ± 22 $-9 \rightarrow 89$	-35 ± 19 $-85 \rightarrow 3$
30–39	35 ± 11 $14 \rightarrow 55$	44 ± 20 $-13 \rightarrow 79$	-36 ± 22 $-97 \rightarrow -2$
40–49	27 ± 19 $6 \rightarrow 48$	37 ± 31 $-20 \rightarrow 99$	-33 ± 25 $-109 \rightarrow 9$
50–59	27 ± 12 $6 \rightarrow 53$	34 ± 28 $-15 \rightarrow 142$	-31 ± 27 $-108 \rightarrow 16$
60–	21 ± 10 $0 \rightarrow 47$	42 ± 54 $-41 \rightarrow 180$	-16 ± 31 $-107 \rightarrow 27$

Table Z: 96-percentile ranges of maximal T vector angle (degrees) in males.

Age (years)	Frontal	Sagittal	Transverse
18–29	28 ± 15 -6 → 60	154 ± 18 110 → 184	45 ± 17 13 → 81
30–39	25 ± 17 6 → 48	154 ± 21 96 → 180	44 ± 17 5 → 78
40–49	27 ± 16 5 → 56	155 ± 18 113 → 180	46 ± 17 9 → 76
50–59	25 ± 14 3 → 51	156 ± 21 98 → 181	46 ± 20 2 → 78
60–	32 ± 18 10 → 81	147 ± 26 95 → 176	38 ± 25 2 → 65

Table AA: 96-percentile ranges of maximal T vector angle (degrees) in females.

Age (years)	Frontal	Sagittal	Transverse
18–29	30 ± 9 8 → 50	134 ± 26 61 → 178	28 ± 18 -15 → 62
30–39	29 ± 10 9 → 48	137 ± 26 80 → 183	30 ± 19 -15 → 68
40–49	30 ± 16 9 → 56	140 ± 21 98 → 185	34 ± 17 10 → 77
50–59	29 ± 26 8 → 53	140 ± 26 82 → 187	33 ± 29 -13 → 76
60–	38 ± 30 0 → 153	144 ± 22 78 → 180	40 ± 24 -6 → 105

APPENDIX 2

Normal limits of paediatric 12-lead vectorcardiogram

The vector data presented in this Appendix have been obtained from X, Y, Z leads derived from the 12-lead ECG according to the methods described in 3.3.4 and using the coefficients presented in Table 3.3. Data have been derived from 1,782 neonates, infants and children, whose age distribution is shown in the upper part of Table 4.1.

Data are expressed as mean ± standard deviation below which is given the 96 percentile ranges, i.e. 2% of values are excluded at either end of the distribution except when the total number in the age group is small, in which case the 100% range is presented. Angular data are presented with respect to the reference frames illustrated in Figure 2.9.

Scalar measurements from the leads X, Y and Z

Table A   Maximal spatial P, QRS and T magnitudes

Table B   Maximal P, QRS and T vector angles in transverse plane

Table C   Maximal P, QRS and T vector angles in frontal plane

Table A: Maximal spatial P, QRS and T magnitudes.

Age	Max P	Max QRS	Max T
< 24 hours	0.16 ± 0.05 0.09 → 0.25	1.83 ± 0.48 0.95 → 2.76	0.25 ± 0.08 0.08 → 0.41
1 day	0.17 ± 0.05 0.09 → 0.25	1.71 ± 0.43 1.03 → 2.48	0.23 ± 0.07 0.11 → 0.38
2 days	0.17 ± 0.05 0.10 → 0.27	1.62 ± 0.41 0.93 → 2.51	0.25 ± 0.08 0.12 → 0.43
3 days	0.17 ± 0.04 0.10 → 0.25	1.60 ± 0.41 1.00 → 2.48	0.28 ± 0.08 0.14 → 0.43
≤ 1 week	0.18 ± 0.05 0.10 → 0.31	1.53 ± 0.35 0.99 → 2.36	0.34 ± 0.10 0.16 → 0.55
≤ 1 month	0.18 ± 0.06 0.08 → 0.26	1.38 ± 0.40 0.76 → 2.04	0.37 ± 0.10 0.19 → 0.60
≤ 3 months	0.16 ± 0.04 0.07 → 0.24	1.87 ± 0.45 1.17 → 2.95	0.43 ± 0.09 0.28 → 0.60
≤ 6 months	0.15 ± 0.04 0.09 → 0.27	1.70 ± 0.38 1.02 → 2.35	0.44 ± 0.12 0.27 → 0.67
≤ 1 year	0.17 ± 0.05 0.11 → 0.25	1.81 ± 0.48 1.09 → 2.80	0.49 ± 0.11 0.30 → 0.69

Table A: Maximal spatial P, QRS and T magnitudes (continued).

Age	Max P	Max QRS	Max T
1–2 years	0.15 ± 0.04 0.09 → 0.24	1.86 ± 0.49 1.03 → 2.82	0.47 ± 0.14 0.22 → 0.70
3–4 years	0.15 ± 0.04 0.09 → 0.24	2.20 ± 0.53 1.25 → 3.21	0.53 ± 0.15 0.21 → 0.84
5–6 years	0.14 ± 0.04 0.08 → 0.24	2.46 ± 0.55 1.56 → 3.61	0.58 ± 0.15 0.31 → 0.87
7–8 years	0.14 ± 0.04 0.08 → 0.23	2.43 ± 0.48 1.56 → 3.38	0.61 ± 0.15 0.36 → 0.90
9–10 years	0.14 ± 0.04 0.07 → 0.23	2.51 ± 0.53 1.55 → 3.33	0.65 ± 0.18 0.34 → 1.00
11–12 years	0.14 ± 0.05 0.07 → 0.24	2.43 ± 0.52 1.45 → 3.51	0.60 ± 0.19 0.30 → 0.92
13–14 years	0.14 ± 0.05 0.06 → 0.25	2.29 ± 0.59 1.25 → 3.60	0.58 ± 0.20 0.26 → 1.00
15–16 years	0.14 ± 0.05 0.07 → 0.27	2.17 ± 0.61 1.20 → 3.23	0.55 ± 0.20 0.24 → 0.95

Table B: Maximal P, QRS and T vector angles in transverse plane.

Age	Max P	Max QRS	Max T
< 24 hours	22 ± 38 $-42 \rightarrow 70$	-6 ± 108 $-131 \rightarrow 181$	23 ± 69 $-76 \rightarrow 136$
1 day	28 ± 35 $-47 \rightarrow 78$	-10 ± 113 $-139 \rightarrow 216$	-4 ± 68 $-105 \rightarrow 132$
2 days	25 ± 35 $-49 \rightarrow 83$	26 ± 111 $-135 \rightarrow 217$	-32 ± 49 $-92 \rightarrow 92$
3 days	26 ± 31 $-45 \rightarrow 73$	10 ± 99 $-138 \rightarrow 206$	-43 ± 42 $-100 \rightarrow 66$
≤ 1 week	24 ± 33 $-46 \rightarrow 67$	34 ± 88 $-130 \rightarrow 210$	-44 ± 31 $-92 \rightarrow 20$
≤ 1 month	15 ± 36 $-63 \rightarrow 66$	29 ± 89 $-126 \rightarrow 185$	-25 ± 33 $-80 \rightarrow 10$
≤ 3 months	8 ± 37 $-67 \rightarrow 62$	14 ± 37 $-111 \rightarrow 62$	-31 ± 26 $-93 \rightarrow 31$
≤ 6 months	6 ± 33 $-41 \rightarrow 59$	10 ± 44 $-107 \rightarrow 74$	-38 ± 22 $-72 \rightarrow 14$
≤ 1 year	11 ± 34 $-62 \rightarrow 67$	13 ± 38 $-45 \rightarrow 83$	-45 ± 19 $-87 \rightarrow -13$

Table B: Maximal P, QRS and T vector angles in transverse plane (continued).

Age	Max P	Max QRS	Max T
1–2 years	23 ± 36 -50 → 69	-19 ± 50 -110 → 89	-38 ± 25 -83 → 5
3–4 years	20 ± 36 -48 → 76	-28 ± 28 -109 → 27	-22 ± 21 -64 → 16
5–6 years	28 ± 37 -43 → 87	-29 ± 21 -96 → 7	-10± 17 -45 → 23
7–8 years	19 ± 39 -46 → 82	-30 ± 21 -63 → 16	-4 ± 17 -40 → 35
9–10 years	17 ± 37 -50 → 87	-31 ± 30 -62 → 10	3 ± 18 -31 → 43
11–12 years	14 ± 39 -53 → 82	-33 ± 19 -78 → 4	9 ± 17 -21 → 51
13–14 years	10 ± 44 -62 → 90	-32 ± 27 -71 → 9	9 ± 17 -20 → 41
15–16 years	4 ± 43 -57 → 81	-29 ± 50 -93 → 204	20 ± 20 -19 → 56

Table C: Maximal P, QRS and T vector angles in frontal plane.

Age	Max P	Max QRS	Max T
< 24 hours	54 ± 14 27 → 74	79 ± 87 -90 → 208	76 ± 69 25 → 151
1 day	58 ± 16 18 → 78	88 ± 80 -106 → 190	67 ± 39 18 → 135
2 days	58 ± 21 12 → 83	77 ± 81 -71 → 191	62 ± 43 23 → 102
3 days	52 ± 23 -41 → 72	67 ± 79 -68 → 194	54 ± 22 16 → 106
≤ 1 week	57 ± 14 22 → 77	62 ± 65 -46 → 186	51 ± 22 19 → 94
≤ 1 month	54 ± 14 30 → 81	61 ± 68 -19 → 190	42 ± 19 18 → 82
≤ 3 months	56 ± 12 25 → 79	36 ± 25 4 → 135	38 ± 22 18 → 94
≤ 6 months	56 ± 13 26 → 77	35 ± 27 -7 → 105	36 ± 13 13 → 56
≤ 1 year	56 ± 14 18 → 76	31 ± 35 -18 → 97	41 ± 16 21 → 75

Table C: Maximal P, QRS and T vector angles in frontal plane (continued).

Age	Max P	Max QRS	Max T
1–2 years	57 ± 14 5 → 73	41 ± 38 -73 → 151	38 ± 17 16 → 72
3–4 years	58 ± 16 23 → 82	39 ± 23 12 → 127	34 ± 10 18 → 55
5–6 years	52 ± 28 -36 → 82	37 ± 20 13 → 101	29 ± 9 11 → 46
7–8 years	54 ± 22 3 → 75	38 ± 18 13 → 63	29 ± 8 12 → 46
9–10 years	50 ± 25 -21 → 80	41 ± 19 15 → 65	26 ± 8 12 → 45
11–12 years	53 ± 22 -26 → 85	39 ± 17 15 → 72	28 ± 8 9 → 42
13–14 years	44 ± 41 -91 → 81	41 ± 17 13 → 74	28 ± 8 12 → 46
15–16 years	50 ± 34 -90 → 82	47 ± 32 11 → 181	28 ± 9 11 → 47

Index

149

Index

Index

Index